Playfulness and Dementia

Bradford Dementia Group Good Practice Guides

Under the editorship of Professor Murna Downs, Chair in Dementia Studies at the University of Bradford, this series constitutes a set of accessible, jargon-free, evidence-based good practice guides for all those involved in the care of people with dementia and their families. The series draws together a range of evidence including the experience of people with dementia and their families, practice wisdom, and research and scholarship to promote quality of life and quality of care.

Bradford Dementia Group offer undergraduate and post graduate degrees in dementia studies and short courses in person-centred care and Dementia Care Mapping, alongside study days in contemporary topics. Information about these can be found on www.bradford.ac.uk/acad/health/dementia.

also by John Killick

Creativity and Communication in Persons with Dementia
A Practical Guide
John Killick and Claire Craig
ISBN 978 1 84905 113 2
eISBN 978 0 85700 301 0

other titles in the series

Leadership for Person-Centred Dementia Care
Buz Loveday
ISBN 978 1 84905 229 0
eISBN 978 0 85700 691 2

Risk Assessment and Management for Living Well with Dementia
Charlotte L. Clarke, Heather Wilkinson, John Keady and Catherine E. Gibb
ISBN 978 1 84905 005 0
eISBN 978 0 85700 519 9

The Pool Activity Level (PAL) Instrument for Occupational Profiling
A Practical Resource for Carers of People with Cognitive Impairment
4th edition
Jackie Pool
ISBN 978 1 84905 221 4
eISBN 978 0 85700 463 5

Enriched Care Planning for People with Dementia
A Good Practice Guide to Delivering Person-Centred Care
Hazel May, Paul Edwards and Dawn Brooker
ISBN 978 1 84310 405 6
eISBN 978 1 84642 960 6

For Sitar
With Much Love
John

Playfulness and Dementia

A Practice Guide

John Killick

Foreword by Professor Murna Downs

Jessica Kingsley *Publishers*
London and Philadelphia

'Small boy' by Norman MacCaig on p.17 has been reproduced with kind permission from Birlinn Books.

Claire Craig has kindly given permission for the quotes on p.21–2.

The quotes from Whitehead (2008), in Chapter 4, have been reprinted with kind permission from Julie Whitehead.

The dementia monologues, in Chapter 6, have been reproduced with kind permission from James McKillop, Nancy MacAdam and John Killick.

The quotes from Knocker (2000) and Knocker (2010), on p.37–8 and 61–2, have been reprinted with kind permission from Sally Knocker.

The photographs in Chapter 9 have been reprinted with kind permission from Rende Zoutewelle.

The photographs in the central colour plate have been reprinted with kind permission from Michael Uhlmann (www.uhlensee.de).

First published in 2013
by Jessica Kingsley Publishers
116 Pentonville Road
London N1 9JB, UK
and
400 Market Street, Suite 400
Philadelphia, PA 19106, USA

www.jkp.com

Library of Congress Cataloging in Publication Data
A CIP catalog record for this book is available from the Library of Congress

British Library Cataloguing in Publication Data
A CIP catalogue record for this book is available from the British Library

ISBN 978 1 84905 223 8
eISBN 978 0 85700 462 8

Printed and bound in Great Britain

For Sue Benson

*in gratitude for all her work for people with
dementia and their supporters over the years as
Editor and Conference and Congress Organiser*

Contents

Foreword

John Killick must be one of the best known poets working directly with people with dementia. Indeed he has pioneered this approach to amplifying the voice, views and experience of people with dementia. I have had the pleasure of hearing these poems on many, though never enough, occasions. In *Playfulness and Dementia*, Killick turns his attention to the central importance of play to the well- being not only of people with dementia but also those who care for, and about, them.

There is no doubt that dementia is associated with profound loss and sadness. What is perhaps less well known is the humour, silliness and playfulness which many people with dementia continue to enjoy. Indeed, many family carers and practitioners have told me that one aspect of caring that they find most rewarding is the opportunity for shared fun that they continue to have with people with dementia. It is timely that *Playfulness and Dementia* be part of our series of Good Practice Guides.

In many ways play is the ideal vehicle for opening the many closed doors experienced when living with dementia. It provides all of us with permission to leave behind the rational, planned and cognitive and embrace the creative, spontaneous and relational aspects of life. In *Playfulness and Dementia*, Killick seeks to inspire a 'new generation of playful practitioners' by providing an overview of the nature of play and innovative approaches, complemented by accounts of playfulness in practice. I have no doubt that he will do so.

Professor Murna Downs
Series Editor of Bradford Dementia Group Good Practice Guides
University of Bradford

Introduction

This book is in part an act of atonement for a misjudgement. In 1997, Tessa Perrin published an article in *The Journal of Dementia Care* entitled 'The puzzling, provocative question of play'. I was provoked, and wrote a letter that was published in the magazine. In it I completely dismissed her thesis that play is essential to well-being and stated:

> Advocating 'play' with people with dementia is splashing around in the shallows and ignoring the deep water that stretches to the far horizon.

In the years since I have come to completely revise this opinion and now maintain that playfulness has much to contribute to the mental and physical health of those with the condition.

This is a judgement I have come to partly through my own experience, but also from encounters with others: people with dementia, family carers and professionals, some of whom are represented in these pages. The book is in two parts. The first part is made up of chapters on the nature of play and what it has to offer people with dementia, and accounts of various practices that have proved innovative and successful. There is also a chapter contributed by Sarah Zoutewelle-Morris on the playful approach to art and craft activities. The second part consists of five accounts of playfulness in practice – two from people with the diagnosis, two by family carers who have gone on to volunteer to work with people with the condition, and one from an actor who has a decade's experience of creative approaches using humour; some of these come from edited interviews. I am very grateful to all these contributors, and also to Claire Craig, whose reflections form an important part of Chapter 2. I am also deeply indebted to the German photographer Michael Ullmann for allowing me to include pictures from his wonderful collection on humour and dementia.

It will have become obvious that this is not a book of argument but rather a collection of first-hand accounts and anecdotes, which, taken together, present a working portrait of an important and neglected aspect of dementia. To find those arguments expounded in exemplary fashion, one must turn to Chapter 5 of a book called *Wellbeing in Dementia: An Occupational Approach* by Tessa Perrin and Hazel May, published in 2000. This, so far as I am aware, is the only serious consideration of the theoretical approach to this subject yet attempted. My endorsement does not extend to the development of Piaget's theory of child development applied in reverse to people with dementia that this piece of writing also contains, but otherwise I am happy for my book to be regarded as a practical series of illustrations of what is involved in bringing humour into people's lives. I have tried to avoid giving instructions of any kind but to let the stories speak for themselves; in this way, I hope that a new generation of 'playful practitioners' will be inspired to take this approach further.

PART I

Chapter 1

What do We Mean by Playfulness?

Play is the unfettering of mind and body; it is without purposefulness; it welcomes the unexpected. In children, it is a natural response to the awareness of being alive in the senses, in collaboration with total unfamiliarity with the environment; it is without boundaries and fearless; it is uncensored and tireless.

In the adult world, play has to contend with every kind of obstacle in its path – the perception of childishness by others, and by the self; the idea that it is contradictory to the work ethic; the impression that it is time-wasting; that it is unproductive in material terms; that it enshrines the principle of the abandonment of learning. It also has to break through the barrier of custom and convention, erected by many years of coping with adulthood and society's laws and habits. It challenges tired perceptions and stale procedures.

Yet play is needed at all stages of life. It enshrines so many possibilities: of learning new things about the world and the self; about reinvigorating the body through exercise and the mind through imaginative forays; about positive enjoyment that refreshes the spirit and helps to prolong active engagement; in social groups, it promotes bonding and encourages intimacy;

it is a continual rediscovery of the basic principle of joy in simply being alive.

For the child, play is fundamentally physical – it is almost an electrical charge: many children cannot keep still – it is partly excitement, partly testing the boundaries of possibility, partly the elation of seeming to be able to move in so many directions at once. In age, play has largely gone inward. With the body less able to perform feats, to accept challenges other than those posed by the most minimal exertions needed to perform basic tasks, play has necessarily to be largely that of the imagination. Just as children explore language through play, older people can experiment with words, and if and when that means of expression deserts them, there is still the possibility of finding an outlet through non-verbal means, involving facial expressions, gesture and the many uses of the hands to support meaning, from mime to drawing, painting and modelling.

Stephen Nachmanovitch opens his remarkable book *Free Play* with a definition of the Sanskrit word 'Lila'. As well as 'play', it carries the meaning 'delight and enjoyment of this moment'. He distinguishes 'play' from 'game'. The former is unconstrained whereas the latter has to conform to a set of rules.

On another occasion he remarks:

> This is the evolutionary value of play – play makes us flexible. By reinterpreting reality and begetting novelty, we keep from becoming rigid. Play enables us to rearrange our capacities and our very identity so that they can be used in unforeseen ways. (Nachmanovitch 1990)

If we examine both the observations contained in the quote in the context of dementia, we can see an immediate relevance. It is often said that, because of memory loss, people with dementia are forced into a continuous present of experience, and, if this is so, any opportunities we can give them for filling those moments with 'Lila' are to be welcomed. The spontaneity of play is a key component of momentary living, which discriminates it from all those other activities that rely upon an accumulation of past occasions for their significance.

It is also often said by family carers (and sometimes by people with dementia themselves) that dementia forces upon people a process of coming to terms with changed circumstances (a reinterpretation of reality?) and some see this as an attack upon the self, so perhaps play can alleviate some of these characteristics at least temporarily, and may even have the potential for a more permanent contribution to positive states.

Here is a poem that seems to embody some of these ideas:

'Small boy'

He picked up a pebble
and threw it in the sea.

And another, and another.
He couldn't stop.

He wasn't trying to fill the sea.
He wasn't trying to fill the beach.

He was just throwing away,
nothing else but.

Like a kitten playing
he was practising for the future

when there'll be so many things
he'll want to throw away

if only his fingers will unclench
and let them go.

(Norman MacCaig 2005)

This poem can be considered a profound and cogent expression of the idea of play, and the contrasts between the small boy's and the adult's attitude towards it. The small boy, like the kitten, is playing physically, and learning at the same time ('practising for the future'). The adult, however, is set in his ways – he can't 'throw away' any more: it is all in his mind that the need is there but he can't 'unclench' his fingers. The impulse to hang onto things has overcome the one to let go. Many people with dementia, though, have already lost so much that this may make it easier for them to 'unclench' their fingers and indulge in play once more.

Chapter 2

To Play or Not to Play?

When you enter a nursing home lounge and see all the residents ranged around the walls facing inwards and not towards the windows and the outside world or each other, with perhaps a TV set on but no one watching it, or a radio blaring out, you are faced with a dilemma in an acute form. Surely most of these people would welcome a playful interlude? Or are there individuals who would prefer to be left to their internal musings, or to slumber, rather than be called upon to respond in any way? And how would you discriminate between them?

I have been on residential units in which an artificial sense of jollity is created with bubbles, balloons and squeakers. This may be acceptable for the occasional party, but the attempt was being made to keep it going for all the residents' waking hours. Surely this would prove wearisome for all concerned, and constitute an unthinking insult to those who could not choose to be elsewhere?

Between these two extremes must lie a happy medium of sufficient stimulation without overload. This must apply to all forms of activity – not just play – indeed, to communication in general?

Usually, if you wish to communicate with other people, you approach them and ask them if they are happy to have an interaction with you. On the basis of their response (primarily verbal), you then proceed or withdraw. With people who are experiencing communication problems, sometimes of considerable severity, it may be difficult to ascertain their reaction. If your object is to issue an invitation to play, the reaction may be wholeheartedly positive, as expressed non-verbally. Where little response is detectable, this may mask an affirmation or indifference or rejection. Do you press the case for play, hoping for an eventual outcome that justifies your boldness, or should you leave individuals to their isolation in the hope that this is what they have chosen? We must always be aware of the power imbalance between those with the condition and those who would seek to continue or establish relations with them. There can be no clear answers to a predicament such as this. We must judge each situation on its merits and hope that we have got it right.

This is the first ethical dilemma in this area of which I am aware, and it is in the nature of the condition that it confronts us. The second one is not so fundamental but is thrown up by the way Western civilisation has developed and how this has an impact on people with dementia. Just as the emphasis on intellectual ability and the consequent devaluing of qualities of emotional honesty and creativity work against people with dementia in our society, so does the overvaluing of seriousness and responsibility result in the rejection of playfulness as childish and scorned when displayed by adults.

This is a learned response, but it is imbibed in our childhood. Of course, young children will play, whether encouraged or not, but if parents and other relatives play with them, then normal maturation will occur. Socialising with other children, inside or outside the family, encourages this tendency. But the education system gets hold of us at an early age, and gradually solemnity sets in. The protestant work ethic soon begins to hold sway. Play is regarded as something for small children, and punished where it interferes with serious study. Only in certain areas of the curriculum such as organised games is it permitted, and this is a narrow, strictly regulated channel. In addition, children observe the demeanour of adults around them, and see their play-denied lives as the models to which they must aspire. By the time the children have reached maturity, play as direct experience has almost disappeared from their lives. It survives in disguise in the proliferation of passive entertainments and hobbies, some of which hark back to childhood enthusiasms.

So to advocate play for people with dementia is to run counter to an established culture and is almost bound to provoke adverse comment in others and even active opposition. This is an ethical argument that has to be won before play with people with dementia can be wholeheartedly embraced.

Claire Craig (personal communication 2012) is an occupational therapist who values play but has met with this kind of opposition, which forced her to question her own values:

> One of the loveliest things is when a person with dementia invites me to join them in play. Suddenly I am stepping into their world. Because this world might be unfamiliar or less familiar I find myself more attentive. I notice more. I start to see things from different angles. Initially there might be a twinge of self-consciousness before I get into the flow – a sense of forcing myself to see things from their perspective – but then I manage to cast off self-consciousness and become lost in the moment.
>
> Yet others are always trying to burst this bubble. 'But it's not real, Claire. You are confusing people. People require reality, truth.' 'That's not the point,' I say in a defensive tone, 'the point is it's play, it's imagination, it's discovery. It's not about reality, it's about learning to be another.'
>
> I feel judged, in trouble. Yet my objection to their arguments is simple. We all play. Granted this might be more sophisticated – it might take the form of a game or a computer animation, or a team-building course.

We are drawn to play, it's a form of leisure. So why, if it is OK for me to play, is it not OK for someone to play because they have a label of dementia?

I was once accused of being demeaning to a person because I joined her in sitting and stroking a toy bunny she had on her lap. A member of staff walked past and said, 'How disgusting, I bet she wouldn't let her mother do that!' It didn't matter that the person was completely engaged in the activity, that she had chosen to take this from a reminiscence basket the week before and kept it with her, or that it prompted her to talk about the rabbits she had owned as a girl – it was impossible for the staff to see past the fact that it was a toy. Of course I was devastated by the comment. The last thing I would ever want to do to someone would be to demean them. I hadn't felt that – I was enjoying the rabbit as much as her, and probably for exactly the same reason. However, it burst my bubble, made me feel inhibited the next time I came alongside her.

I must have been upset because I asked a very wise person with dementia about the experience who said, 'I like nursery rhymes. They make me feel safe. Perhaps the other people were sad because they felt on the outside.' I think this is true. People who reject play, who label it as demeaning, only view it from the outside and never really understand it. This is probably even more pronounced in places where the dominant paradigms of science and health prevail. Here knowledge, certainty and control are valued – those very factors that are almost the antithesis of play.

Fortunately there are many instances of play being valued by family carers and professionals, and the rest of this book consists of examples of stories and projects where its positive powers have been successfully harnessed.

Chapter 3

What People are Already Doing

Some people, trying to find ways to help people come to terms with their dementia, and indeed to help themselves to make their caring situation more satisfying, have stumbled upon play as the opening of a magic door to shared and increased well-being. One such is Bernard Heywood, who in a book published in 1994 provides a kind of journal of his regular visits to Maria, a neighbour with dementia living on her own.

In the first of three extracts he describes in general terms the nature of his discovery:

> I've...devised a new aid to good relations and her well-being by making her laugh. This is achieved by indulging in antics – acting, gesticulating and walking in odd ways as one would with a child, or indeed like a real comic doing a routine. So it's been very helpful.
>
> These antics remained helpful on and off for a considerable time, and my repertoire increased. It included wearing one or two comic, or comically arranged, hats, and odd ways of dressing. Just as she could sometimes cry excessively, Maria could also laugh excessively. It was nice, though, when this happened. (Heywood 1994, p.116)

In a later entry, Heywood provides a more specific example of one of his 'ploys':

> After tea Maria became very cheerful and frequently laughed (some of it was over-reaction). This was chiefly due to one of the new tricks I've devised. One of my old bedroom slippers has a sizeable hole at the big toe and I stick things through it – a pen, a toothbrush, a tube of toothpaste and so on. It looks comic and when she catches sight of it – for I don't draw her attention to it, though I put my foot where she's likely to see it – it amuses her mightily. This particular item was one of those malleable brushes you use to clean sink pipes. It's a trick that has come in handy, though I don't like to overexcite her. (p.124)

Heywood finds that looking at photographs and paintings with humorous content often provokes merriment, and watching Laurel and Hardy and Charlie Chaplin films raises Maria's spirits. He also makes up comic songs to sing to her.

When another neighbour, Mrs Wright, comes on the scene, the opportunity presents itself for comedy antics involving all three of them:

> Mrs Wright came to give me a break. It was a big success. As usual, she got on very well with Maria and there was much laughter. This laughter often arose from looking together at scrapbooks that I had made for her, or postcards, and playing with things. It would sometimes culminate, on my return, with me cautiously putting my head round the corner of the door and then quickly withdrawing it (with various permutations on that general theme) while Mrs Wright feigned alarm with Maria. (p.128)

It is impossible to prescribe specific games that might appeal to everybody. A sense of humour remains a personal attribute, and what will make one person laugh may occasion a stony-faced response in another. It will be a matter for you to experiment with and build up a repertory of playful approaches. All I can give are examples from real-life situations that have been found to be effective. In almost every instance, improvisation, being prepared to 'go with the flow', will be necessary.

Here is Sunny Vogler, whose mother had dementia, with her friend Koren, rising to the occasion in just this way, as described in her book published in 2003:

> Mom and I sat outside drinking margaritas and playing Rummy-O with the tiles. Koren came by to see what all the laughter was about and joined in the fun. She asked, 'What are the rules to this game?' I answered with a smile, 'There aren't any. Just drink your margarita and play.'
>
> Each of us took turns picking up tiles and placing them down in any order we chose. Mostly the game consisted of putting tiles down in a group of the same color or the same number. At some point I would shout, 'Mom, you win!' We would laugh and drink and start the game over. Finally Mom said, 'I think you're letting me win.' Grinning and pretending to be shocked at her accusation I asked, 'What makes you think so?' She laughingly replied, 'How can I keep winning when I don't know what I'm doing?' After that, Koren and I took our turns yelling, 'I win!' (Vogler 2003, p.51)

On another occasion Sunny and Koren introduced a puppy to the household. That proved the catalyst for Mom to invent her own playful ritual, which kept her actively involved for long periods:

> From the moment Koren and I first brought her home, Mom pretended not to love the puppy and Chloe kept out of her way, unless they were playing 'the game'. It went like this. The glass sliding door at the rear of the

house was usually left open during the day. Without breaking her travel pattern, Mom would open the front door and tell Chloe to go outside; Chloe trotted out. Mom would continue through the house and Chloe would race around the side to the back patio and wait. Before Mom made her turn at the back door, she would stick her head out and holler, 'Come on in, puppy.' Chloe would come bounding in, happy to be playing the game. Then Chloe would wait while Mom made the entire circuit and opened the front door again. This would go on all day, neither tiring, until Chloe was side-tracked by a lizard or by the kids playing in the street. (p.77)

A third example from the same book illustrates the power of play to enhance relationships:

One late afternoon, we decided to go out to eat. I said, 'I'll shower and change and you get dressed too.' Twenty minutes later, I walked out of my bedroom to behold my mother pacing around the house stark naked. The shock factor alone kept me from laughing. We stood there looking at each other – she smiling and me shaking my head, puzzled at this new development. OK, she got it half right. She took off the house dress, but couldn't decide what to wear. Wrong. I took an outfit from her closet and laid it on the bed saying, 'This will look nice. Put it on so we can go out to eat.' With fingers crossed, I left the room. Less than a minute later, she appeared, still nude. I chuckled as I turned her around and pushed her back into her bedroom. 'Mom, you're going to catch a cold going out to dinner like that!' We kept laughing as I dressed her.

Standing on the porch as I locked the door, she stopped me and said, 'I'm glad you're here.' I held her close and nose to nose replied, 'Me too, or you'd probably get arrested.' We continued walking to the truck, howling with laughter. (p.78)

Jim Connor is an Australian carer, and in his book *A Funny Thing Happened on the Way to the Nursing Home* he tells many stories of situations in which humour ameliorates or resolves dilemmas. The chapter entitled 'Tea with the duchess' is the most elaborate of these. One evening, when Jim and his wife Norma settle down for the night, she suddenly orders him out of bed because 'The duchess is coming to have a cup of tea with me.'

Rather than arguing with her, he goes along with this fantasy and they get the house ready for the distinguished visitor. Norma instructs Jim: 'Don't you make any of your cracks about the royal family. Those aides of hers don't have a very good sense of humour, and...' She stopped speaking and drew her open hand expressively across her throat.

The duchess, of course, doesn't appear, and Jim has to find a way of compensating his wife for her disappointment. This is what he does:

> Suddenly an idea dawned on me; there was a light coming from a telephone box across the road. I ran to it and dialled our number. I knew Norma wouldn't answer the phone... When I heard the telephone ringing in our house, I left the receiver of the public phone dangling. I ran up the steps to our phone which was playing its merry little tune in the hall. Picking up the handset, I began a sorrowful conversation with a crestfallen look on my face (I was fast becoming an actor). I put the phone down and turned to Norma:
>
> *That was the duchess. She asked me to convey her apologies for all the trouble she has put you to, but her car has broken down and she is unable to make the journey. But she will get in touch with you and come to see you another time.*

She suggests you have a cup of tea and go to bed. (Connor 1997, pp.4–6)

Norma is satisfied with this explanation. Improvisation and a sense of humour have saved the day.

Robert Breckman (2002) in an article entitled 'Julie smiled with eyes overrunning with laughter' is a carer with a similar message:

> When I tell a joke she laughs. I am safe in telling it to her again since she will not have remembered it. She still laughs at the silly jokes we had before she became ill. She laughs when reminded of her mother's reprimand of some 50 years ago: 'Shut your mouth and eat your food.' When she says something, albeit incoherent, and laughs, I laugh too. I repeat the last word and we sit together as I gently punch her to get and continue the reaction of mirth.
>
> Physical jokes appeal to her. I fall over her feet and she literally screams with delight and tries to trip me up again. And when Brian, our pug, kisses her face she falls about – especially when I follow suit. I make dirty innuendoes and she reacts with gobbledegook and we both act like giggling, naughty schoolchildren.
>
> When I greet her I play hide and seek behind a door and she laughs uncontrollably. I make dirty noises and she does likewise. And when I say I am going to steal a biscuit from the tea trolley, she joins in the fun. Returning with a digestive sends her into paroxysms of glee. I put my finger to my lips to indicate secrecy and she follows suit. And when I give the thumbs up she mimics me. (Breckman 2000, p.6)

Other ways Breckman identifies as eliciting positive responses are miming in various settings, and, less obviously, sneezing. He is a man with the unfortunate tendency, when a sneeze afflicts him, of repeating it a number of times. This itself provokes hilarity in Julie. When *she* sneezes, he embarks on a comedy routine that involves tossing his handkerchief about and wiping all the objects around. He sums up his philosophy of playfulness in the following words:

> All this may seem petty but playing the fool and being inventive keeps me sane. And if she laughs whilst others around me gaze uncomprehending, who cares? She laughs, and that is worth more than its weight in gold. (p.6)

There are many examples of the inventive use of language by people with dementia elsewhere in this book. Notable ones from a carer are provided by Elizabeth Cohen (2003) in *The House on Beartown Road,* her autobiographical account of single-handedly looking after her small child, Ava, and her father with Alzheimer's:

> While we are eating the chilli, Daddy bursts with wit and spontaneous humor. When Ava steals his fork, he calls her a 'forklift'. When she climbs onto the table and grabs the salt shaker, pouring white grains all over the floor, he says, 'At least we know she's a mover and a shaker.' (Cohen 2003, p.153)

It would appear from these examples that Cohen's father is aware that he is being funny. But Cohen also manages to appreciate his unconscious humour:

> There is an undeniable beauty in the way he is losing language, the way he substitutes different words when he cannot find the one he wants. He calls toast 'the singed bread', and apples 'the crackly, magnificent, sweet ones'. Sometimes he calls me and Ava 'the beautiful big one' and 'the beautiful little one'. (p.55)

The bond between the small child and the old man provides many opportunities for play:

They often laugh together. She has a plastic alligator with a mouth that opens. She likes to put her finger in its mouth and say, 'Oh no!'

It cracks them up.

Then he puts his finger in the alligator's mouth. 'Oh no!' he says.

She laughs so hard I worry that she will fall over or not get enough air and faint. (p.59)

Cohen sums up what she has learned from caring for individuals at both ends of their life span:

I think that a sense of humour must be hidden in a box very deep in the brain, where diseases have to search for it. Maybe this is an evolutionary tactic, to keep people going. (p.27)

John Bayley, in the first of his three books about his wife Iris Murdoch, seems to reach the same conclusion:

Humour seems to survive anything. A burst of laughter, snatches of doggerel, song, teasing nonsense rituals once lovingly exchanged, awake an abruptly happy response, and a sudden beaming smile... Our mode of communication seems like underwater sonar, each bouncing pulsations off the other, and listening for an echo. The baffling moments at which I cannot understand what Iris is saying, or about whom or what... can sometimes be dispelled by embarking on a joke parody of hopelessness, and trying to make it mutual. Both of us at a loss for words. (Bayley 1998, pp.56–7)

Chapter 4

Bringing Play to the Person

The use of improvised drama to connect with people and arouse their own sense of playfulness is proceeding apace, and in this chapter I shall illustrate a number of examples in practice.

Clowning is one form that the provision of playfulness in institutions has taken, and, as in so many instances, Tom Kitwood, the psychologist, saw the potential before most other people. In a report on a conference he wrote the following:

> ...the work of two 'relational clowns' (much more friendly, playful, gentle and empathic than the typical circus clown) who seem to be able to evoke remarkable responses from people who are depressed or severely withdrawn. The presence of the clowns itself excites attention and their gestures and movements evoke an immediate response, often without the use of words. (Kitwood 1998, p.11)

Individual clowning projects have taken place in a number of countries, including America, Canada, Holland and Australia, and their effectiveness is still being written up and evaluated. Some of these are offshoots of the 'Clown Doctors' movement that has been so successful in children's hospitals.

Korey Thompson in America is a clown doctor, and she has written vividly of what she calls 'Therapeutic Clowning' with people with dementia. She describes how she attempts to initiate a session as follows:

> The essence of 'Therapeutic Clowning' for me is a non-verbal Question and Answer Dance that proceeds at the pace set by the patient. As the clown, I will ask the first question by inviting a patient to 'come out and play today'. The patient can answer 'No', and I will accept their answer. If I sense confusion or uncertainty in their answer, I may respectfully 'ask' a second time by doing another short action by myself that they can observe and respond to if they wish. If they want me to go away, I will. I can also come back on another day when the answer might be a 'Yes'. (Thompson 1998)

Once a session is under way it may take many spontaneous forms, but a feather duster is a prop that plays a significant part. First it is used to dust furniture. Then Thompson uses it to dust parts of her own body. When a person's curiosity is aroused, Thompson transfers the brushing movement to parts of the person's own body. Gradually a joint playfulness is established. Here is a description of how she copes with a really difficult challenge:

> One time when I was visiting a woman with severe dementia, I had tried the ever faithful feather duster routine to no avail. She remained fixed on staring blankly into space. I was not able to make any eye contact or receive any response from her at all even though I was going very slowly. The nurses on the ward indicated that she would not be able to respond and that I should try to 'chat' with someone else. For a while it seemed like they were right, but I thought I'd blow some bubbles as I waved goodbye to leave the woman surrounded by their gentle joy.

I got out the Bubble Bear and blew a cascade of bubbles. One of the bubbles popped a couple of inches in front of the woman's cheek. She turned her head and looked straight at me, smiled and said, 'You blew a bubble, didn't you? I could feel it.' I heard the nursing staff murmuring in the room. I nodded my head, 'Yes' and blew a couple more cascades. She smiled and even laughed a little and watched the bubbles. In a few moments, I felt it was time to go, and waved my hand to say 'Bye-Bye'.

She replied by singing out, 'Nighty-night! Sleep tight! Nighty-night! You know I was sleeping tight when you came. Yes, I was asleep. Nighty-night! Sleep tight!', and she waved a frail hand to me as she left. It was a real moment! (Thompson 1998)

Elderflowers is a clowning project based in Edinburgh that has been very successfully going into hospital wards and stimulating responses from individuals for a decade now. It is an offshoot of a Clown Doctors programme run by an organisation called Hearts and Minds. Those who deliver the programmes are professional actors trained specifically to work with this client group. It was decided at the outset not to go down the line of full dress and make-up as clowns, which might prove distracting or even frightening to those to be approached. Instead, a working compromise was reached, with suggestions of the clown but also signs of normality. The red noses are clown-like, but there is no specific costume. The actors carry cases full of props, which can be brought into play as they make relationships and develop situations that bring out the humour of the participants.

Here is an extract from an account of a session. Ian and Maria are the actors, Ann is an occupational therapist who works on the ward, and Bob and Frank are resident there:

Suddenly Ian, Maria, Ann, Bob and Frank find themselves in a circle, arms round each other, dancing.

Nobody seems to know how it happened: they were all seemingly carried away by the impetus of improvisation that was set up. Bob begins to sing, making up the words as well as the tune. Some of the lines go like this:

'We can dance all the way.

All the way along the road.

And what can we see?

Absolutely nothing!'

'Absolutely nothing!' becomes the chorus, chanted lustily by all. Then Bob sings:

'I hold the lie!

I'm the biggest liar!'

A red nose falls off and lies there in the middle of the circle. 'Play the ball!' Frank shouts, and a frantic game of football ensues. Then he shouts again, 'But we haven't got a centre half!' Everyone falls about laughing. (Killick 2003)

A feature of this episode is that Frank and Bob are the initiators throughout. I recall that after the session was finished (it was lunchtime) Bob was reluctant to leave, but eventually was persuaded to join the others. About ten minutes later he returned. 'I don't want to leave my friends', he said. I see this as an example of how playfulness can quickly build relationships.

Clearly Bob's response to the session was very positive. But playfulness can also accommodate a range of feelings. I returned to the hospital the following week to talk to some of the residents on the ward who had taken part in the sessions:

He [I] showed Vera a photograph of the two actors, and reminded her of their names, Honey Bunch and Sweetie Pie. Then he produced a red nose from his pocket similar to the ones they had worn, and to the one she had put on on that occasion. She took it from him and put it on. 'I think the noses are good', she said. Then, handing it back, she told him, 'Put it away. I wouldn't like it to be harmed. Till they come again.'

She pointed to the photograph: 'They're beautiful children. They must be full of fun. They don't make me feel sad. I'm always very pleased to see them.'

She went on to point to Ian: 'Someone he loved very much might have died, so he's sad too in a way. They're definitely actors. I talk to them and they talk to me nicely. They play with me, chase me, and I pretend to run very fast. They make me laugh, but only as an act. I like to join in, in very small bits, correcting them. They are my friends. I like them very much.' Then she sang the whole of the Scottish song 'My ain folk' and commented, 'I see them as funny and sad and friendly.'

This exchange took place in a busy corridor. It was typical of the responses I got from participants. Some were less articulate than Vera, but even those whose verbal ability was severely restricted managed to respond positively to the prompts. Janet, who appeared only able to manage to shake or nod her head in answer to his questions suddenly said 'mouthorgan', which was an instrument used on the day. After he had put his props away, she spoke all in a rush: '*I'm* not acting, *they* are. I quite like them. They're not too fast, no bother. I watch them all every time, I'm just myself.'

Another participant, who appears in the DVD *Red Nose Coming* comments, 'I find them funny, yet I don't find them funny.' The ambiguity expressed here is not uncommon. I believe it is symptomatic of the richness of the experience on offer.

Maria, who was Ian's partner in the exchanges described, tells how one of the staff told her one day that some of the patients had recently been moved from the ward that

Elderflowers had been visiting regularly, and she was worried about them because there were no activities on the new ward and they had really enjoyed the interactions. She wanted the actors to continue working with them but didn't know how to arrange this. Maria, Ian and the member of staff to whom they were talking decided to go and visit the ladies and meet the staff to effect an introduction. Maria takes up the tale:

> We went in and before we had time to properly introduce ourselves both ladies came 'running' towards us! 'There you are… I can't believe it…let's dance… I'm crying… you came to see us!' They hugged us, joked and laughed. The staff stood there with both eyes and mouths wide open. (M. Oller, personal communication 2002)

Elderflowers provides one kind of interactive theatre, 'Ladder to the Moon' another. The latter is a London-based company that works in care settings. Their 'performances' also usually involve two actors, but they arrive armed with a plot and props. The story may come from Shakespeare or a film classic, but they invite residents to take some of the main roles. The potential leads are approached and addressed perhaps as 'my lord' or 'my gracious queen' with a bow and the proffering of a crown. The reaction soon tells if the offer is accepted. The people chosen are usually delighted, and grow in confidence and stature as the drama is acted out. They are by no means the most obviously able people, as is shown by this comment from an activity co-ordinator:

> The lady who played the Queen is deteriorating daily; and today we saw a different person: she was attentive, involved and appropriate; she came in on cue, she exceeded everyone's expectation of her.

Chris Gage, the company's director, comments on the process:

> With a nod and a wink we acknowledge that we are all playing together, we can do anything we like, everything is accepted, everything playful. (Benson 2009, p.20)

In another article (Graty 2008) Gage makes the following assertion, one which he acknowledges has come to assume ever greater dominance in the company's aims:

> It can change staff members' perceptions of what people are capable of and what is possible within the home.

Sally Knocker, who is a member of the Ladder to the Moon's board, comments:

> By being spontaneous and responding to audience members who want to join in the actors truly involve people. People with dementia can be particularly prepared to be playful because they can be more disinhibited and this is sensitively handled. (Benson 2009)

The use of props to provide a stimulus is well developed as an improvisation technique, and Paul Batson, a drama therapist, comments in an article on one aspect of this:

> I have a collection of hats. I buy them from charity shops or borrow them from our local amateur dramatic society. Some hats have a specific purpose such as a builder's hat or a military hat. Others, especially ladies' hats, tend to indicate the kind of occasion when one might wear them such as an everyday hat or one for a special occasion like a wedding.
>
> I have often been surprised at the level of energy that develops in a 'hat session'. I also note that many people are more proactive than normal and seem to be able to make choices more naturally than they

usually do. They soon start to interact with each other, commenting on one another's appearance. Compliments are often forthcoming and individuals can gain the attention of the group. Having a number of mirrors available is essential. It is also important to be aware of and sensitive to anyone who may feel a little self-conscious in such a session.

A hat session can be developed in a variety of ways depending upon the abilities within the group. It may be possible for people to talk about why they chose a particular hat or name an occasion when they might wear it. Memories are often triggered and patients recall events in their life associated with hats. Some might be able to take up a pose appropriate for a hat, e.g. directing the traffic in a policeman's hat. This might even lead on to a brief role play as clients get into a character that they associate with a hat. I well remember role playing with a gentleman who was wearing a builder's safety hat; he had a wonderful time telling me off for my shoddy workmanship. (Batson 1998, p.21)

Sally Knocker offers a vivid example from her work in a care home:

Patricia, a self-contained Irish woman with dementia, is offered a beret during a session with hats. She unexpectedly rises from her chair, puts on the beret with a flourish, and moves across the room on an imaginary bicycle ringing her bell vigorously and saying 'Excusez-moi!' much to the amusement of other residents. She enjoys the attention and does a bow at the end of her performance. (Knocker 2000, pp.4–5)

Although there is a spontaneity here, there is also a social awareness, a sense of an audience, which can be a component of playfulness.

Laughter Yoga is a method that has been tried with some success by practitioners. It was developed by Dr Madan Kataria in 1995. It is based upon the idea that children laugh uproariously and easily but adults lose that ability as they go about their serious and increasingly complicated lives. The theory is to simulate laughter in the hope that it leads to the genuine experience of merriment; this is called 'fooling the body'. Dr Katarina then merges this with the practice of Yogic breathing.

Caroline Coulman describes her experience of using the Laughter Yoga approach:

> I have been working as a self-employed Activity Co-ordinator since 2006, following a number of years working in care. I have added Laughter Yoga to the programme, working with a number of care homes in Shropshire and parts of the West Midlands. The sessions have been run with staff and service users and carers and I've even run a session with a team of senior managers. Some approach the sessions with initial scepticism, but those who give it a go come out with a lift, ideal for starting the day and preparing for life's challenges. Laughter Yoga can certainly help to lift the mood and get the positive endorphins flowing. (Coulman 2012)

Julie Whitehead is another Laughter Yoga practitioner. She was invited to run a session for 12 people with dementia by the Croydon branch of the Alzheimer's Society in October 2008. She describes the event as follows:

> The session was gentle and playful with many of the exercises done seated, but some movement was encouraged to get the energy flowing and a sense of connection across the group. We did some brain gym exercises, played with laughter sounds, drew

self-portraits with our eyes closed and laughed and greeted each other in a playful way. (Whitehead 2008)

And she offers the following accounts of the feedback she obtained:

One lady does not see the purpose in getting up in the morning if she is not going to go anywhere or see anyone – so she just stays in bed. After the laughter session this lady said 'laughter is the most wonderful thing in the world!' She also said 'laughter is the reason.' …

Another lady drew comparison with what she usually feels like – isolated, lonely and that every day is the same. She said 'You need to laugh so you can "forget your troubles". It is healthy to do this. It's amazing what laughter does.' …

Another of the group has very bad back troubles, and does not always want to come to the meetings – but I didn't hear her complain about her back at all, and she made a real effort to get involved. …

There was also a strong feeling that it was good to laugh within a group, as they like to contribute something and help others to laugh too. This made them feel useful to each other and connected, which gave them a good feeling and a sense of purpose. One lady said 'you start laughing and everybody joins in.' …

It is worth remembering that this group are sometimes reluctant to join things – perhaps because their memory problems cause them to feel embarrassed, unconfident or shy. A couple of the ladies needed a great deal of encouragement to come to the group, but they were very enthusiastic after our session on Thursday to come again. This in itself speaks volumes! One lady said 'I'm so glad my sons encouraged me to get involved, I just love it!'

I am not aware of many other attempts to bring Laughter Yoga to people with dementia or of a proper evaluation of the method having been done, but until then it can certainly be considered as a possible approach for those wanting to increase the well-being of this client group in a potentially stimulating manner.

A research team from St Andrews and Dundee Universities has developed a conversation support system and a set of innovative games for people with dementia and their carers. The Computer Interactive Reminiscence and Conversation Aid (CIRCA) provides touchscreen access to thousands of reminiscence items – photos, songs and film clips – which can be enjoyed by the person with dementia, along with a carer or relative. Both participants can explore the system easily via the touchscreen. Every now and then (typically several times per session) a long-term memory is triggered for the person with dementia, which their conversation partner has not heard before.

The CIRCA software takes over from the carer or relative the responsibility for keeping the conversation rolling, and both participants can relax and enjoy exploring the reminiscence material and having chats based on what memories are stimulated. One of the research team's discoveries is that personal material is not needed to stimulate memories, and, in fact, generic material from archives does a better job of prompting a wide range of responses from users.

The team has also developed a number of interactive games accessed by touchscreen, which they have called Living in the Moment, since they can all be enjoyed without the need for an intact working (short-term) memory. These games have proved enjoyable as a shared activity, and in many cases a person with dementia has been able to interact with them on their own. The games developed so far include games of skill and creative activities.

The instances given in this chapter are all targeted, time-limited and professional, and there is certainly a place for this.

Not everyone can aspire to this level of stimulus for their loved one or those in their care, but I believe there is much to learn from these strategies that can be applied on the smaller scale of daily life.

Chapter 5

Funshops
Portrait of a Project[1]

This chapter is an account of a piece of work I did with the Scottish Dementia Working Group in 2010. This is an independent organisation of individuals based in Glasgow but with a membership spread throughout the country. It is a campaigning group and also gets involved in innovative projects. The original idea was for me to work with a small number of individuals in one centre, using improvisation and humour as a way in to performance. While this, with the Glasgow group, led to the writing of monologues (see Chapter 6), demand quickly grew elsewhere for a rather different approach, and I put together a new kind of workshop in four centres that met monthly over a nine-month period based in Alzheimer Scotland branches in the north-east of the country.

I had anticipated working with seven or eight people in one place, but I actually worked with a total of forty-four people and eighteen staff across the four centres; these latter were all employees or volunteers of Alzheimer Scotland, who enthusiastically joined in the sessions. Their support contributed immeasurably to the spirit of the occasions, gave

---

1   This chapter is based on an expansion of two articles (Killick 2010, 2011).

them some new insights into what was possible, and was of mutual benefit with their clients in the relationship building that occurred.

It may be asked what qualified me to run such an activity? The fact is that I studied drama at college, in my later years taught drama in further and adult education, and was particularly keen on improvised approaches. More than one play that I produced was invented by the actors before being formalised into a text. When I embarked upon the project in question, I could see the possibilities of drawing on this experience in a fresh context. I had also been involved in the early stages of, and written about, the Elderflowers project in Edinburgh (see Chapter 4), where pairs of trained actors enter a dementia unit with the aim of stimulating responses from the participants. This had convinced me of the power of playfulness in dementia settings. That said, running these Funshops proved a steep learning curve for me.

The benefits of Funshops

First of all, Funshops provide an opportunity for people to relax in a carefree state of mind. Time and again people say that they are freed up to say and do things spontaneously. It's a relief to let go and enjoy, within limits, the freedom that the various exercises and sketches give them, and they also appreciate the opportunity to enjoy other people's release of thoughts and feelings.

Second, there is the laughter that predominates in these sessions. Seeing the funny side of things consistently over a period of time is a respite from confronting changes that may be occurring in people's perceptions and relationships. It reminds them of a powerful characteristic that they all have in common. But it is also the case that it is much easier to laugh in a group than it is on your own.

Third, there is a sense of community engendered. It is noticeable that, however reserved or isolated a person may appear at the outset, once the session has begun this soon begins to fall away. There is usually at least one individual who may be experiencing a degree of disinhibition that may have been caused by their condition, and this person becomes the focal point from which hilarity can spread outwards. I heard the comment a number of times that there seems to be an irresistible force in a group 'which draws you in'. Thus a significant bonding occurs, which is strengthened at every meeting. In one group a man came to me at the beginning of the session and apologised in advance for his lack of a sense of humour. He came back to me at the end and complained that the laughing involved had made his sides hurt!

Liberating effects

Most of the exercises and sketches I devised involved people being themselves. The encouragement of playfulness in each individual is initially a matter of providing opportunities for people to call upon the reserves of humour that are available to them in carrying out their daily lives.

An extra dimension of this is when someone is asked to play with someone else, perhaps someone very different from themselves. This can have a surprisingly liberating effect. In one of the centres I visited a man who was clearly of upright character, and had been contentedly married for most of his adult life, but who took the part most convincingly of a two-timer. He must have astonished himself, because coming out of role he was at pains to assure his companions that he was really clean-living. We can only speculate as to the psychological power involved in, if only for a few minutes, donning the mantle of another.

Comments by participants

Some of the characteristics of the sessions are reflected in comments made to me by different people afterwards:

I wouldn't miss this for the world. It has such a friendly atmosphere. I surprised myself what I was able to do as the interviewer.

I love the atmosphere. Nobody singles you out. We're all in this together.

It's not just being silly. It's being serious. There's something serious behind this. I sit at night and think about what has been said. And it helps.

I enjoy it very much, because it's meeting friends, and it's nice to talk to people, all people who are suffering the same as you from Alzheimer's in varying degrees, and doing all sorts of things, and knowing that you can.

When I come along usually I don't know what to do at first but gradually you are drawn into something, and that's good, it's going into our minds. It's seeing other people, how they are living, where they are going, the kind of things they enjoy and so on. And you sometimes find something – oh I would like to do that too – so you add another piece of information to your body and your mind, and it's worthwhile.

About Alan

Here is a more extended example of how the Funshops have benefited one individual:

On the first occasion the group met, Alan came but his body language suggested great reluctance. The session began with coffee and introductions. He described himself with reticence and modesty. He stated, 'I'm here because of my wife. I don't want to be here. She made me come. She thinks it will be good for me. I have never been to any social event since I was diagnosed with this thing.'

I did my best to make Alan feel welcome. Despite his protestations, I included him in all the exercises and sketches. In one of our brief chats, he vouchsafed to me that he was an amateur painter. I asked him if he would bring some photographs of his paintings to the next session, but I wasn't sure he would even attend.

On the occasion of our second meeting, Alan arrived a quarter-of-an-hour before anyone else, and settled down to talk to me. It was obvious that he was pleased to have a one-to-one chat. However, when the other members arrived, he greeted them and immediately started showing them his photographs and describing how he had come to do individual paintings. He took part in the exercises more readily than on the previous occasion, but he still maintained that he was there under duress. I think we now all saw that this had become more like a comedian spinning a line rather than a genuine complaint. I thought up a special sketch for us to do together. I put him in charge of the improvisation: he was the artist and I was the client commissioning him to paint my portrait. As my demands grew ever more grandiose, he kept a straight face and accepted all the absurd conditions imposed. Finally, he turned to the rest of the group and commented, 'I do not accept this commission.' They all fell about with laughter, and his timing had played a significant part in this. Afterwards I reflected that, taking the session as a whole, Alan had spoken more than any other participant.

At our third meeting, Alan was again early and showed enthusiasm to interact with the others as they arrived. He played a full part in the exercises and sketches. We had ten minutes to spare at the end and I asked the group, 'What shall we do?' Alan immediately stood up and declared, 'I want to say something.' He spoke for the full ten minutes. He said:

When I first came here I didn't want to come. My wife sent me. But I found everyone so friendly and it wasn't difficult to join in. This is only my third visit, but my attitude has completely changed. And that applies to things outside as well.

He went on to describe in detail how he had only wanted to shut himself away and not see anybody. Now he was actively going out to meet people and talking to them, and things felt a lot better for him.

Afterwards I had a conversation with the development officer who organises the sessions. She said, 'I have never seen such a positive change in any client in such a short time.'

What happens in Funshops

From the time when I taught drama in colleges I had a fund of ideas for workshop exercises to use in these sessions, and I put these together with some techniques of the great Brazilian practitioner Augusto Boal, founder of the 'Theatre of the Oppressed'. In trying these out, adaptations and fresh techniques came to me on the spur of the moment. Eventually I had a repertoire that worked – that is, created a great deal of spontaneous humour. I have since tried these out with other groups in different settings and found a similar positive response to the invitation to engage in organised fun activities. Here are some of them.

Saying hello and goodbye

I always begin and end sessions with these activities whether the participants know each other or not. They constitute an invitation and also indicate closure. It is most important, when people are being asked to drop their guard, to set boundaries in which we all operate. The activities consist of saying hello (or goodbye), establishing or using names, and engaging in a physical expression of togetherness (shaking hands, a kiss, a hug, even a little dance – whatever seems most natural).

Since I insist that everyone greets everyone else individually, walking around the room as they do so, this can take several minutes, particularly if it is not the first occasion on which the group has met. Saying goodbye can take even longer, because people want to stay and talk. However, it is important not to cut these rituals short – they are crucial components of the bonding that occurs.

As a sign of the commencement of the Funshop, and that I am the facilitator of the event, prior to the greetings exercise I don an elaborate colourful waistcoat. It could be a hat or a red nose but I have chosen the waistcoat as a symbol of play and a sign that playfulness can begin. It provokes many comments, at the time, and at other times too, and soon is generally recognised as a special garment that makes everyone smile with anticipation or satisfaction as they remember what kinds of things it leads to.

Smelling a flower

Everyone imagines a flower in their hand, which has a beautiful or an unpleasant scent. They take a deep breath of its perfume, and express their appreciation of it (ranging from ecstasy to disgust) in the way they expel the air.

Laughter infection

In pairs, individuals try to make each other laugh, but without speech or touching each other.

Talking gibberish

Partners converse without using intelligible language. (On the surface this might appear one of the more problematical exercises, but I have found that it is just as releasing and reassuring as the others.)

Statues

Again in pairs, one is the sculptor, the other the statue. The sculptor may mould the model into whatever expressive shape he or she chooses, and the statue has to hold that position until the facilitator gives the word. Then they change roles.

Group sculptures

This is a more elaborate version of the previous exercise. Depending on the size of the group, one or two or more sculptors are chosen, and they then choose a number of participants to make a more complex arrangement of interacting figures to express an idea or state of mind.

What has changed?

In pairs, partners study each other's appearance intently, looking at dress, posture and facial expression. They then turn back to back and each makes a slight adjustment in their appearance. When they turn to face each other again, they have to identify the adjustments made.

Mirror images

In pairs, with one at a time leading, partners attempt to follow each other's movements. This is a non-verbal game, and taps into one of the most powerful of communication techniques.

Mexican laughter waves

Everyone stands in a line and attempts the bobbing movement that constitutes a Mexican Wave often practised in crowds, only this time the movement is accompanied by laughter. Since the sound of laughter is infectious, once the laughing begins it soon catches on until everyone is joining in.

Grandmother's footsteps

Based on a children's game, this begins with one participant in the corner of the room, and the others gathered in the opposite corner. The solo person is facing the wall, and when the word is given the others silently move forward. The person may turn round at any time, and, if anyone is caught moving, that person is out. The solo person then faces the corner again and the process continues. The winner is the one who touches the solo person first, and that person then occupies the place in the corner. This is a competitive game, and I have found that some people respond to it with particular determination. It proves highly popular with every group with which I have played it.

What's the object?

For this the facilitator needs to have selected three or four unusual objects to bring along that are particularly interesting from the point of view of touch. Two contestants sit side-by-side with their eyes closed or blindfolded and their palms upturned in their laps to receive the objects. The first object is examined by the first contestant and then passed to the other. The object is then removed, the contestants open their eyes and each in turn is asked to describe the object and perhaps identify it. During this whole process, the other members of the group observe but keep silent. I have found that the degree of concentration shown is often astonishing. It could be seen as a rather testing situation for some people, but if the atmosphere is kept light-hearted then a great deal of merriment can be created. Objects that I have used include an eggcup, a book reading-light, a novelty tape-measure, castanets, plastic columns for decorating a wedding cake and a hand puppet.

Accusation and defence

One partner of a pair accuses the other of an imaginary crime or misdemeanour, and the other has to defend him- or herself. This roleplay has worked well, with everyone participating, and occasionally with one pair performing and the rest of the group as an audience.

Chat show

This is one of those exercises that arose spontaneously and was so successful that it has been repeated many times. In an extended form it can be a standalone activity. One person is chosen as host, and then has the task of choosing which people are to be interviewed and on which aspects of their lives. This can either be played straight or treated as a send-up of the TV format. Taken seriously, everyone learns a great deal about each other in a short space of time. The rest of the group act as an audience and clap and laugh in the appropriate places. (I should add that clapping is encouraged in Funshops at every possible juncture, as a celebration of people's talents and personalities.)

Nine of these 12 activities do not include words at all, so the Funshop is very suitable for those who are experiencing problems with verbal language.

I consider that the techniques used here are capable of considerable development. I have not used costume, props, music or mime to any degree, and I am certain that puppetry has real possibilities.

Chapter 6

The Dementia Monologues

These began as an offshoot of the Funshops (see Chapter 5) and were developed at the Glasgow branch of the Scottish Dementia Working Group in 2010. Members of the group wanted to write and read their own pieces of writing on the subject of dementia but using humour to put their ideas across. Over half a dozen monologues were created, all of them collaborations between an individual and me. All the ideas came from members of the group and I helped to shape the finished pieces. When it came to performance, memory problems prevented the participants from speaking their monologues, so a compromise was reached whereby they read them out. A video was made of four of the monologues, one of which was a new one, entirely composed by its author; this did not especially involve humour, so it is not included in this chapter. Two of the other three are included, plus one that was not filmed because the person was unable to attend the session; it is therefore presented anonymously.

The themes of these three monologues can be loosely described as coping with problems, taking a proactive approach through promoting an active lifestyle, and obstacles to the exercise of memory. Each takes a different approach to presenting its topic, but what they all have in common is demonstrating what Agnes Houston observes in Chapter 11, 'If you have a problem, you solve it with a sense of humour', or, to put it a different way, the perspective that playfulness gives you helps you to see your problems in a whole new light.

Stand-up

Is there anyone out there knows me (*peers at audience*)? Is there anyone out there I know?

Well I'm James and I've got multi-infarct. So let me tell you what it's like to have this mysterious condition.

First thing is, it doesn't affect the way I dress (*clothes are on back to front*).

And you can't tell I've got it by speaking to me. By the way, where are we? What is this place? Where did I leave my car? How do I get back home from here?

I admit you can tell by some of the strange things I do: cars are a speciality. One day I put washing-up liquid in the oil sump.

And if you're a passenger of mine you have to be prepared for a bumpy ride – I keep hitting the kerb.

One day I went round and round a roundabout, looking for the right exit. The right exit was a service station, because my wife was bursting to go to the toilet. Eventually I took the road back onto the motorway, in the direction from which we'd come. A sign read 'Next Services 37 Miles'!

If you're travelling behind me, you'll know it by the way I keep slowly veering from side to side. I don't seem to be able to keep a straight line. I'm not drunk. But try telling that to the traffic police!

Actually the truth is, I lost my licence. Well the DVLA took it away. So now I go everywhere by public transport. I have a bit of a problem with fares. So I count out the money and put it in a small plastic bag before I go. At the start I took the exact fare for getting there, but I forgot I needed the same amount for getting back. It was a long walk home – five miles!

Don't send me out shopping, because I'll come back with some useless object or other. When I get home I can't remember why I bought it. The charity shops are full of items I've purchased and had no use for.

I tend to stay awake at night and sleep through the day. I've invented a word to describe this – I call it MUTONOXDIES. Can you think of a better one?

I hope you're not beginning to feel sorry for me. Despite a few drawbacks, I still enjoy living and meeting dedicated people who look after me.

And I know a few people up and down the country who would willingly change places with me – they're all in graveyards! (James McKillop)

Everything in the garden

'So what's wrong with me, doctor?' I asked. 'You lack vitamins in your body,' he said. 'Eventually your mind will be affected. Like leaves falling from a plant, your mental faculties will shrivel and fail.'

I was alarmed. 'What can I do to ensure some more fruitful years?' I asked. 'I prescribe Baby Bio at your root twice daily. Then your stem will be strengthened and a green old age will be assured.'

Well I set about it at once. I swept all the decaying matter from my life, planted out my faculties in neat rows, and mulched them in vigorously. I feed them faithfully night and morning, prune them regularly, and give any slugs that dare to come near short shrift.

And now you see me in my harvest time. My branches are overloaded with fruit. Here, pick one, have one, there's more than I can eat. All that discipline, that regular effort, has paid off. I am self-sufficient. I dine on my own produce.

I hardly dare consider the consequences if I had lost the plot, and let it be overtaken with weeds and thistles. My simple message to everyone is 'Grow Your Own!' (Nancy McAdam)

Lead me to the Memory Clinic

A funny thing happened to me on the way to the Memory Clinic – I couldn't find where it was!

I asked all sorts of people, and I got some funny answers, I can tell you.

One lad directed me to HMV – he must have thought I said 'the Melody Clinic'. Well, he was only trying to be helpful.

A man thought I was being clever. He

pointed to my head – 'It's in there', he said. 'That's where you keep your memories.' 'I know that,' I said, 'but where do you go when you keep losing them?' 'The doctor,' he answered. 'Oh, I've been to him.' 'And what did he say?' 'He sent me to the Memory Clinic!'

A lady took me to the Lost Property Office at the bus station. I said, 'It's not like I've lost my purse or my bus pass. How can I ask them to look for my memories?' 'Well, they're just as important, aren't they? They're personal to you. And if you've lost them, someone may have found them.' I could see the sense in what she said but I couldn't bring myself to ask the man behind the counter.

Another lady very kindly offered to take me to A & E, but I said, 'They won't be able to help me – I've broken memories, and they can't mend those.'

I ask you, how are you expected to find a Memory Clinic of all places? I looked on the street maps. Nothing. I looked at the signs around the town. Town Clerk's Office – yes. Rubbish tip – yes. No Memory Clinic.

I know what I'll do. I'll make myself a badge – 'I'M A GOOD FORGETTER'. Then perhaps people will come to *me* asking for help!

Chapter 7

Home-made Humour

Clearly playfulness and humour are not the same thing: the former encompasses the latter. And verbal humour is only a part of that concept. Nevertheless, for many people with dementia, especially those for whom language still carries important messages, verbal humour is an essential instrument for warding off negative feelings and helping to keep everyday life on an even keel. This chapter is simply a little anthology of things that people have said to me in my role as a writer (hence the nature of one or two of the quips). It includes remarks on the significance of humour for one or two individuals. The quotations are offered without commentary, but the message they are intended to convey is one of cheerfulness, hope and the cherishing of gifts that people with the condition have given us.

Spending my time? I never earn any!

Is it one o'clock yet? That's shock, horror and murder time! I mean 'The News'*!*

Up to three tons my licence. And now I can't even ride a bicycle!

I've got financial cramp. It's a very well-known condition.

I don't know why people say I'm living with Alzheimer's – Alzheimer's is living with me!

I've got an eye for the men but I didn't put it there!

I had a bath this morning and I felt like a ship-wrecked mariner!

We are still looking for the wonderful piece of medication that will do the job, but in the meantime we need to learn some new songs and some new jokes.

See her, poor hen, she's never been taught to watch television!

If you write down my winks, I'll tell you where you can put your notebook!

I've never sat an exam – there was no ink in the inkwell.

Here's another John. John the Baptist. He'll have to watch his head if he is!

I roar with laughter at people, and they laugh at me. But I don't know any jokes. It's all home-made humour. If it fits, I say the phrase. Sparsmodic. I can laugh and like it.

I became a house builder. The tea making was the mainstay of the building. The building work was quite secondary.

'Write on, write on to victory' – there's a quote for you!

Now don't start laughing or they'll think you're a policeman, that's for sure. It's the notebook: they'll think you're taking statements. If anybody asks me, I'll tell them you've been promoted Detective Inspector.

Chapter 8

Playfulness in the Moment

Sally Knocker trained as a drama therapist, and has brought her improvisatory skills to a variety of care settings. On one such occasion she was caring for Mrs Hamble, a 96-year-old, very frail lady with advanced dementia, who spoke little. It was a fine day and she decided that taking her for a walk in her wheelchair would be a good idea. What happened next she describes in her own words:

> I went with Mrs Hamble to a small local park where leaves were falling from the trees. Sunlight was catching the beautiful array of autumn shapes and colours – oranges, yellows, browns, greens and in-betweens. Mrs Hamble was still fast asleep. I suddenly had a childish impulse (a great asset in dementia care!) to run through the leaves. So I ran kicking them in the air, lifting my arms up high to catch a falling one, enjoying the crunchy sound of contact with those at my feet and the air and sunshine on my face.
>
> Gradually Mrs Hamble's face started to lift from her slumber as she noticed my movement and energy. She started to smile and then called out with great animation, 'Run, RUN!' In that moment, the wrinkled 96-year-old face became transformed – awake, alert,

alive! It was as if she had been transported in time and was six years old again in her mind and in her heart running in the leaves alongside me. Through watching another in that moment, she was able to leave behind her weak body and tired mind to find a place that was light and fun and free again. (Knocker 2010, p.80)

Here Sally Knocker was demonstrating playfulness by example, and, although physical participation was impossible for Mrs Hamble, she was caught up in the moment and shared the air of exhilaration.

Sometimes language can provide the spur. In another anecdote from Sally Knocker's experience it is a line of poetry that sets the creative juices flowing (Knocker 2010):

I was walking down a corridor with a woman called Muriel and we looked out of the window at a glorious summer sky. I said to her, 'It's a beautiful blue' and she replied, 'But it hasn't a hood!' It took a moment but suddenly I felt jubilant as I REMEMBERED THE REFERENCE...to the A.A. Milne poem 'Vespers' and we then proceeded to recite it together with great glee. We ended up skipping down the corridor with our sense of achievement at recalling the whole verse:

If I open my fingers a little bit more,
I can see Nanny's dressing-gown on the door.
It's a beautiful blue, but it hasn't a hood.
Oh God bless Nanny and make her good...

How easy it would have been to just see Muriel's reply to me as confused or meaningless when in fact it was an invitation to share a favourite poem from both of our childhoods.

As one of a series of meaningful anecdotes set in an Australian facility, Barbara relates the following:

One warm spring day, Reg was sitting between his wife and daughter in the sunshine, the gentle breeze lightly blowing his silver hair. He continually leaned over backwards and pulled leaves off the camellia bush behind, crunching them up in his hands and dropping the pieces on the ground. His wife said that he used to play the gum leaves very well as a young man when she first met him. His daughter went off around the street and brought back a range of leaves from different gum trees.

With a big grin, Reg placed them carefully in his lap and felt each leaf. He selected one and placed it between his two thumbs and began to blow. The thin squeaky noise of 'Waltzing Matilda' could be made out from the sound.

His wife's eyes filled with tears. Reg said something like, 'I was a young'un out there in the red and those others told me about it and we did it and they went down and it was done all the time…'

Big tears ran down his wife's cheeks as she said that she had not heard him talking like that for years. It seems that, before he was 20, he had worked on a station property in central Queensland and the Aboriginal stockmen had taught him to play the gum leaves. (Naughtin and Laidler 1991, p.153)

Sometimes unexpected singing and movement can occur. In the following example, the relationship appears to have been the stimulus but the person with dementia then took over and verbalised and danced his sense of joyfulness:

I had had conversations with Sandy over many weeks. They had always been very downbeat, and I thought he might have depression as well as dementia. One day I heard him speaking with the head of the unit. She asked him if he was feeling comfortable and he replied, 'What pain ever goes?' On another occasion he said to me, 'I'm all muddled up. I'm hopeless. I'm useless. I'm nearly crying.' The day before the remarkable happening I shall describe in some detail, he said to me, 'I'm not like you. You're a really brilliant chap. You can see and do everything. I'm just an ordinary character, not like you.' I replied, 'You're a really nice man, Sandy.' He said, 'Nice man's not enough on its own. Far better to be nice man *and* what you've got.'

The following day Sandy greeted me with handshakes and smiles. The unit was built on the courtyard system with a garden in the middle. Sandy set off around the corridor, which eventually brought him back to where I was standing. He was running and jumping as he completed the circuit and singing at the top of his voice. It was a kind of operatic aria, though I couldn't quite catch the words. When he was level with me again, he stopped and said, 'It's time we did some work. To work and sing.' And then he was off again. The next time he came round, he stopped and sang to the group of staff and residents who had gathered:

He's got the love.
He's one of the best.
He knows what to do.

Yes, John, terrible tie –
Get rid of the blasted thing!
But you're a wonderful man.

He's got love. He's got it.
He's got beauty, that loveliness.
Now you can see it again.

He's got love. Just take it
When you feel you need it.
No need to take it right now.

That good man, lovely man,
That Christian man –
He is beyond us all.
He's one of the nicest chaps
I've ever heard sing.
We can't sing the way he speaks.

So don't stop, don't rush,
Don't stop being beyond us
Because that's what we need.

This was a kind of recitative. Then he was away again, singing another aria and dancing. When he came around for the third time, he motioned to me to join him, which I did. I didn't know the words or the music but I too improvised, and we hopped and skipped hand in hand all the way round the square. We stopped for breath and Sandy turned to me: 'What are we doing here?' he asked. 'I have no idea', I answered. 'Why are we doing this?' This time I replied, 'Because we want to!' We both roared with laughter, embraced, and he danced and sang on alone. He kept up this high energy activity for a further 20 minutes, before, exhausted, coming in for his tea. (Knocker 2000)

There is a pattern to be discerned in much playful activity with people with dementia, and that is that the stimulus is often supplied by another individual before the playful potentialities are released. One could almost see this as a *Sleeping Beauty* syndrome. The person is awakened by a word or a gesture or a pattern of movement (or a kiss) and then she is away on her own, sometimes as an almost unstoppable force. We need to be aware of what a significant role we can play in this process.

Chapter 9

Even a Few Scribbles

Sarah Zoutewelle-Morris

Sarah Zoutewelle-Morris has made an outstanding contribution to the development of art and craft activities with her book Chocolate Rain. *She lives in Holland, but is a significant presence on the British scene. Here she reflects on her experience of the playful approach to creativity, and suggests an activity that can bring pleasure to all.*

When I accepted a position as an activity director at a psychiatric care home here in northern Holland, I'd worked with people with dementia before, and counted on my long experience as a healthcare artist to transfer easily to a new situation. However, I was unprepared for meeting a population largely non-conversant with the arts.

Naturally, there were a few 'arty ones' who went to the activity room for closely directed handwork sessions. But my job was to 'activate' those left behind in the lounge, and, at first, no one could be coaxed to have anything to do with visual art activities. As soon as my art supplies appeared, the people disappeared. Holding a brush, cutting or folding paper, modelling clay, etc. were all viewed as too childish by the majority of the residents.

Over the next five years, working with people in all stages of dementia, my ideas about what an art activity (or any activity for that matter) is, underwent radical changes. The insights and practices gained on this journey are documented in my book, *Chocolate Rain, 100 Ideas for a Creative Approach to Activities in Dementia Care* (Zouteurelle-Morris 2011). As well as being an activity resource book, it is a creative manual designed to support anyone working with people with dementia to become more creative, spontaneous and playful in their approach.

In this case, success in reaching people eventually came when a degree of trust and familiarity had been established. I let go of my preconceptions and my planned activities; instead I gently entered their lives each week as a familiar person coming to spend meaningful time together. I took my cues for what to do from the person and situation I found at that moment. The best days were the ones when I was able to communicate my genuine excitement about some material or technique I wanted to share, and that enthusiasm sparked a response.

Being an artist helped because I was comfortable with, well, being uncomfortable! The creative process is full of wrong turns and failed results. One learns to keep experimenting until things rearrange themselves into a new configuration. This new situation (or painting, poem, concerto, etc.) is often a *result* of those 'failed' results and 'wrong' turns, and could not have been foreseen at the beginning of the process.

Usually, I entered the lounge after lunch and met ten drowsy individuals, each unoccupied and each isolated. At the end of the afternoon, many of those people would be actively engaged doing something around a table, and family and staff would be either looking on or participating. There was talk and laughter and social activity, all centred around a few simple materials, or even just a topic for discussion.

Regarding painting and other art activities, there will always be one or two people who make visually pleasing work, but I don't consider this the goal of the activity. Shifting the emphasis away from 'good' or 'right' *results* to the *process of making* precludes failure on everyone's part, including the person leading the activity. And it invites all kinds of playful experimentation that can result in real surprises and even intriguing artwork.

In evaluating the results of an art activity, we tend to look first for realistic imagery or at least a harmonious whole. But I try to help caregivers (and activity directors, friends, family, etc.), and the person who made the work, to take a slightly different perspective. Even a few scribbles on paper can be found worthwhile for their own sake if looked at a certain way. Assessing the work from an *abstract* visual art angle allows the results to be appreciated based on many different kinds of qualities: rhythm, emotional power, variation, stroke, colour, shape, weight, etc.

This mode of perception is not familiar to most people outside the arts, but it can be learned. Caregivers and other medical staff could take a class in any area that teaches how to progress from an idea to a tangible result using a creative skill – for example carpentry, book binding, creative writing, metal working, garden or interior design, theatre, clowning, drawing, etc. In the United States there are medical/art programmes whereby doctors in training receive a course in art appreciation. By learning various ways of seeing, their diagnostic abilities are enhanced. Skills gained this way are increasingly valued as important supplements to purely scientific, intellect-based thinking.

The arts seem to almost *require* a playful state of mind in order to experience every moment freshly and keep creating. Creative people learn by experimenting and improvising. They come to trust the process they are in whether or not they know where it will lead. And they develop a feeling or intuition for when to stick with the original plan, and when to let it go and flow with what is happening at that moment. These, and a light, playful attitude towards a bit of healthy chaos all help in communicating with people with dementia.

And, especially in cases of advanced dementia, they aid one in navigating a reality based on a different logic from one's own.

There was a group around a table engaged in making a collage together. A man from another floor came in, sidled up to the table and 'stole' bits of paper. I started unobtrusively leaving him interesting torn and crumpled pieces where he could spirit them away then return for more. This was a legitimate activity for him and a form of non-verbal communication between us.

Approached in this way, an activity is relieved of having to *produce* or *achieve* something. Its worth lies in whether someone is enjoyably engaged and whether they seem to be doing something that has meaning for them.

Even the simplest circumstances can lead to meaningful occupation. One day, looking for an activity requiring minimal means and preparation, I filled a bowl with warm suds. One by one I brought it to each of several ladies seated around a table. Emily 'did the wash', including her doll, its clothes and her glasses; the second woman played with my hands under the suds, then, as I was giving her a hand massage after, reversed roles and gave me one instead; the third woman did the dishes; and Gré, my 'spontaneous friend' and I blew hand bubbles.

In my book (literally and figuratively!), this fulfils many requirements for a meaningful creative activity:

- There was one-to-one quality attention given.

- There was group interaction and a relational aspect.

- Laughter, surprise and silliness were all present.

- Each woman preformed an action with the soapy water that had meaning for her.

There was nothing produced and little achieved, but the activity was successful nonetheless.

A parting word about something like blowing bubbles, which may seem too trivial an activity for adults. It is the *intent* of the leader/performer that will be communicated. If she is genuinely enjoying herself and respecting the activity and the audience, then whatever she does will be received as a playful pastime for adults rather than an attempt to entertain them with a 'child's' activity.

In the end, it isn't the means employed but the simple attention, respect and imaginativeness one brings to the encounter that leads to real engagement.

How to blow hand bubbles

Needed: washing-up bowl filled with warm water, dishwashing liquid.

Procedure: wet your bubble-blowing hand in the water, squeeze a dab of dishwashing liquid in the centre of the palm. Rub it around with the fingers of the same hand. Capture a film of soap somewhere between your first fingers and thumb by forming your hand into an oval and tucking the rest of your fingers in to form a channel (as shown in Figure 9.1).

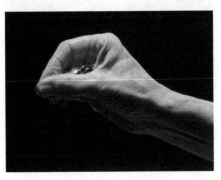

Figure 9.1 Soap film caught in the oval formed by curved fingers and thumb. Credit: Rende Zoutewelle

Blow onto the soap film, forcing it down into and out of your hand – an oblong bubble should form (see Figure 9.2). When it is large enough, pinch it off by keeping your hand in the same position, but closing the fingers, then flick your wrist and the large bubble will float into the air (see Figure 9.3). Your hand should be soapy and wet for this to succeed, so keep the washing up bowl close under your hand throughout to catch the excess suds and water.

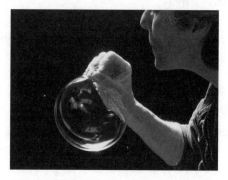

Figure 9.2 A medium large bubble like this should stay intact when 'squeezed off'. Credit: Rende Zoutewelle

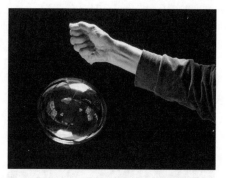

Figure 9.3 With practice, the bubble slides off the hand easily. Credit: Rende Zoutewelle

Like any skill, it takes practice. Be sure to use plenty of dishwashing liquid, and find the balance between blowing too hard and too lightly.

Separating the bubble from the hand is a bit tricky, but, once you master this, washing up (bathing, household chores, etc.) will never be the same again. Have fun!

Chapter 10

Taking the Senses for a Walk

Paul Klee characterised the activity of drawing as 'taking a line for a walk'. In this chapter I look at play that gives full rein to all the senses. Of course there are aspects of the subject covered elsewhere that involve appeals to the senses to a greater or lesser extent. Many of the Funshop exercises, for example, are devised to attract this kind of response. But here I am particularly concerned with activities for those with more advanced dementia, for whom the verbal channel is largely closed but the physical and emotional aspects of the human are still available for expressive purposes.

The Snoezelen is a sensory space consisting of various equipment such as fibre-optic lights, bubble tubes, mirrorballs, creating a total environment where colour and image and sound hold sway. Music can have an important role in establishing this kind of ambience. While there are some individuals who find the Snoezelen more of an assault course than a stimulation, others take to it easily and enthusiastically. Kim Wylie (2001), an Australian educator, describes the effect on Kathleen, a woman who had spent most of her life working for an industrial cleaning firm as well as bringing up a family:

> Kathleen arrived at the sensory room accompanied
> by a staff member who had packed all of Kathleen's

soft toy companions into an infant's pram. Surrounded by 20 bears and soft toys, we sat while Kathleen enlightened us about ways to 'burp and settle a bear'. She showed us the best way to rub a bear's back and put it to sleep. 'You stroke it from here right down to here' she wisely told us. Every now and then, she would gently touch her bear and whisper 'there, there little fella, you're a dear little fella.' Her hands, gnarled and arthritic from years of domestic toil, held each soft toy tenderly as she shared with us her maternal wisdom and knowledge.

Throughout the session, Kathleen looked down at us as we sat on the floor either side of her and advised us if we were caring for our toys in the correct manner. When she thought that we were not, she guided us appropriately. If we inadvertently referred to a bear as a 'baby', she corrected us by saying 'you mean the bear'. Kathleen knew that the bears were toys and referred to them as a bear or a doll, or a frog, according to their shape. Nevertheless the bears seemed to be providing her with an essential outlet for her motherly love and affection.

When we were confident that Kathleen was at ease with the environment of the room, we switched on each of the sensory pieces and then sat back, nursing our bears and listening to the music. We sat as three ordinary women, watching the lights in the bubble tube change colour as they rose slowly to the surface, smelling the fragrance of geranium and lavender aromatherapy oils, stroking our toys and enjoying one another's company. Despite the fact that the staff member and myself were both middle-aged, it did not seem to us to be out of place nor did we feel uncomfortable holding and stroking our toys.

Kathleen's playful nature was infectious and at one stage we found ourselves rolling about on the floor, laughing until the tears trickled down our cheeks. Kathleen looked down at the staff member and in between roars of laughter she chuckled, 'you're nothing but a big kid'. Tears of laughter covered her face and ours. We did not need to share temporal or spatial worlds, or to engage in meaningful or rational conversation, in order to enjoy and appreciate each other's presence. (Wylie 2001, p.23)

This description conveys a number of important messages. Most significant is that Kathleen remained in a maternal role, but without the pressures that immersion in that period of her life had brought. Now she could relax into the freedom of play that dementia had brought. Second, she was the dominant person in this scenario, and brought joy to those who accompanied her. Third, she was fully aware of playing, and that that was different from real-life motherhood.

The Woodlands View Day Hospital in Lancaster has developed an initiative that they call 'Woodlands Therapy' (WT) (Pulsford, Connor and Rushford 1999) which also involves a Snoezelen, but alternates this with more conventional play activities, including the use of balls, balloons, party blowers, bubble blowers, dolls, soft toys and microchip-controlled talking toys. They reported mixed responses but:

All people appeared to derive enjoyment from at least some of the play-based activities. For instance, one game of balloons lasted for a full 12 minutes and provided one of the most lively and good-humoured sequences on the videotapes. The dolls and soft toys also proved valuable. One lady became very attached to a battery-operated parrot, which repeated back what was said to it. She asked after the parrot at the beginning of each session and talked to it at length, chuckling at the responses. Another person liked a rather garish fluffy duck, which sang nursery rhymes when its wing was pressed. Most people liked holding a large life-like baby doll, borrowed from one of our children. Best of all was a small battery-operated dog, which walked across the floor. All participants in WT have found it fascinating. (Pulsford *et al.* 1999, p.15)

As with Kathleen in the previous example, there seemed to be the possibility that individuals could hold in their minds the double role that objects played – that of being real creatures and also playthings:

A comment from the person who liked the toy parrot shows that she regarded the parrot in a complex way: 'I like to hear him talk. He tries to say what you say. I have to keep him in mood, because he'll get lazy. It must be batteries or something inside. If I don't talk to him he'll get lazy.' (p.15)

The authors also make an important point about the significance of the uninhibited attitude of the individual carer in creating the right kind of atmosphere for playfulness to flourish:

This was illustrated by an outgoing and bubbly student nurse who facilitated one session, and got a much better reaction from using party blowers than other staff. She brought a greater sense of fun to the activity, people responded with laughter and approving comments – and a great deal of noise! (p.15)

In a remarkable article, Angela Byers (1995), an art therapist, describes working with individuals with advanced memory loss in a kind of 'play therapy' of her own devising. She would provide a variety of materials, sometimes including paper, cloth, small plastic containers, string, wool, sticky tape, gum-strip paper, a pencil, a ruler, scissors, a screwdriver, balsa wood, stones, a sponge, modelling clay and jelly. These would be placed in a random way on a table or tray. A person would be encouraged to handle them, smell them, perhaps even taste them, and arrange them in whatever order or pattern they chose.

Participants would often become absorbed in exploration of these items for long periods, sometimes combining them to make something new or modifying them in some way. At the same time they would often engage the therapist in conversation or be engaged in an internal commentary on an activity. People would sometimes appear to be engaging with an object directly and sometimes to be expressing themselves symbolically. Byers believed herself to be included in the process, which she describes as a triangular relationship with the play area being the third angle of the triangle. She observes that people whose memories are severely impaired lose interest in making marks on paper as in painting, but this is subsumed by the process of playing with the materials for their own sake and finding meaning in this activity.

Sue West (2009), a family carer, has written about how she has designed play objects for her father. When she visited him in the nursing home, she observed how the shape and texture of a handbag strap absorbed him and this prompted her to make him a sensory book from white cards tied with thread. The pages were in bright colours and covered with different textures. Her father had always been a reader, and now he would turn the pages and systematically take the book to pieces. She decided to experiment further and invented 'Fiddlers'. These were pieces of board, with holes drilled in them and colourful shoelaces and pipe cleaners threaded through them. Her father received these enthusiastically and spent long periods weaving and tying with much satisfaction.

Sensory play has many possibilities, and we need to experiment to find the mode that suits the individual.

Pictures of Playfulness

Michael Uhlmann

I saw some of the photographs in the German magazine 'Demenz' and immediately wanted them for the book. The images on the following pages need no captions: they express visually, and more directly, what the text is trying to say.

Michael Uhlmann was born in 1958 in Magdeburg, Saxony-Anhalt, Germany, and currently lives in the Börde district of the city. He works as a freelance photographer, specialising in themes ignored or suppressed in society.

Photography, especially portrait photography, can be a way to facilitate encounters – even if we weren't looking for encounters with people whose presence might be unusual, even unpleasant, yet always allowing for an encounter with oneself as well.

In my photography I try to shift the focus and perspective of the observer. I wish to capture people with dementia who seem to be beyond our limits from a 'demented' perspective, in order to make them once again visible in the eyes of society. At the same time I'd like to sensitize the observer and make him/her more open for possible encounters, and for a view of life from a different perspective – fearless, welcoming and open-hearted.

My photos on humour are part of a larger project called 'Was blelot – Menschen mit Demenz' (What remains – People with Dementia) that I have been working on together with my wife, Petra Uhlmann, for the past nine years. Humour, laughing and joy are all abilities and possibilities that people with dementia do not lose; on the contrary, they are an emotional expression of their affectivity and humanity just as much as fear, hunger and pain. Humour can be a door-opener and an opportunity to communicate – even when cognitive and verbal abilities are limited. This is what I would like to convey with this photo series, emboldening people to tread new paths with people with dementia.

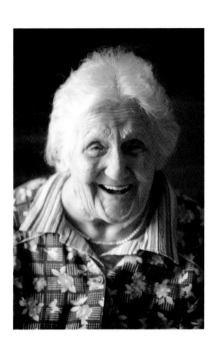

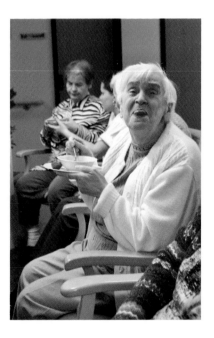

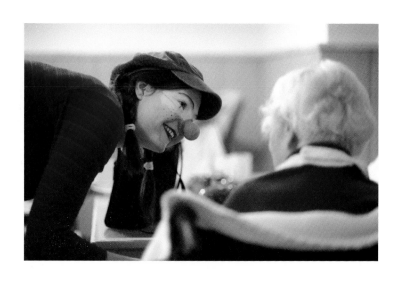

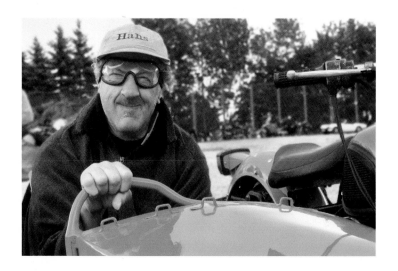

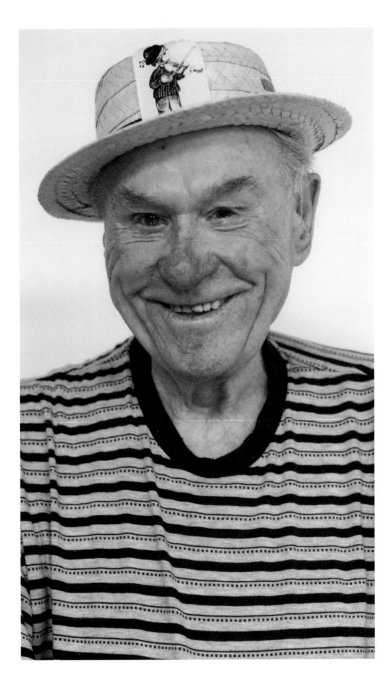

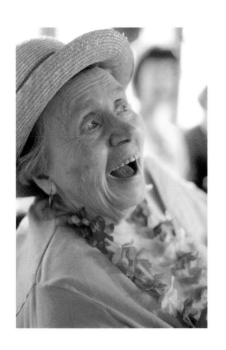

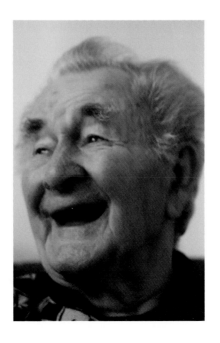

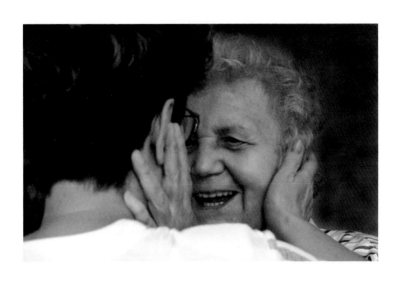

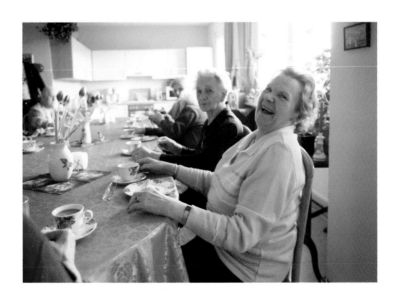

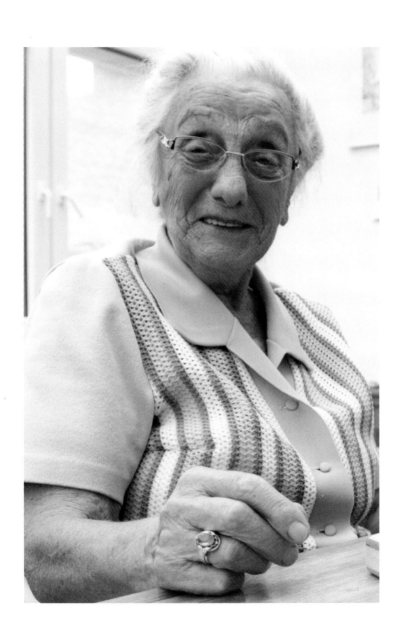

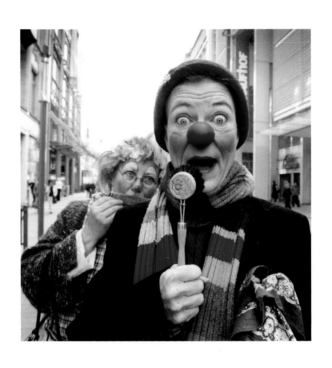

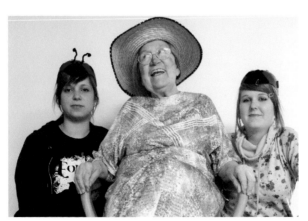

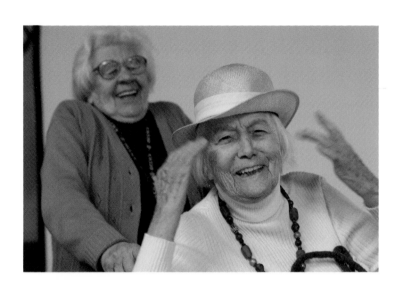

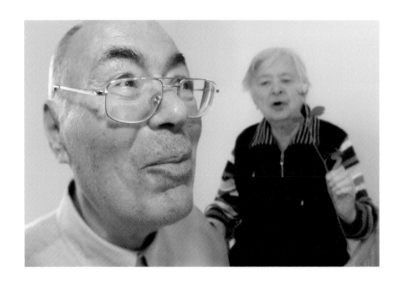

PART II

Chapter 11

A Licence to be Free

Agnes Houston

A significant presence on the vibrant national dementia scene is the Scottish Dementia Working Group; indeed, it has an international reputation. One of the most prominent members of the campaigning group is Agnes Houston. She is tireless in her promotion of the views of people with dementia, and is determined to develop her own creativity, particularly in the visual arts and drama. The latter attitude is reflected in her contribution.

I didn't think I had a sense of humour. I was too busy being serious. Then when I got dementia I was having to focus on myself for the first time in a long time. Suddenly I had to look at myself to see what I could put in place – who was this different Agnes? Eddie and James and the group started talking about humour. Then it was fed back to me that I *do* have a sense of humour; so do my brothers. Then I started using humour as a tool in a lot of things.

I can see the fun in a situation, and I can feel myself smiling internally; then it comes into my face. I can find the fun in a lot of situations that can be quite serious, like everybody else is losing their cool, and I can feel a bit of fun and bring it in, and before you know it people are beginning to be a little more light-hearted. It takes the sting out of a lot of sore situations. There's a lot of humour in the Scottish Dementia Working Group (SDWD) and it's that type of humour. When you're sitting there they might bring up quite a sad situation and then you might get David spilling it into looking at it from a different angle. I realise I had that there all the time.

I'm not saying dementia's not serious. I've just had a serious conversation with my nurse, but tomorrow I'll probably be thinking about it and the dynamic will have changed. When I'm re-telling that, there'll be a lot more humour in it. I'm going to say that it's a licence in a way – a licence to be free, to be me. I think when I got the diagnosis I got permission to be freer, more relaxed, and to be me, relaxed into this person and to accept her.

I found this a total surprise, because before, coming from a nursing background and working for a chiropractor, everything's just so, and regimented if you like, to make the wheels continue in motion, and it's nice to be a wee bit looser and freer and give rein to thinking outside the box.

My dad's dementia has had a big part in my life, and has affected the way I treat my diagnosis, because my dad had a great sense of humour and a twinkle in his eye. I was Ms Practical: 'We'll have to get this done. We'll need to get this sorted. We'll put this in place.' I was a problem solver. And then he told me this story of how when he was with my mum they went on a lot of pilgrimages. My mum had an artificial leg and was in a wheelchair, and my dad was the main carer. Of course he had undiagnosed dementia at the time. She did all the thinking and he did all the doing. My mum said 'Boil the kettle for a cup of tea', and he had to find his way to the kitchen and back again. Well, this was difficult. How he did it was that in the corridor in hotels and other places there are pictures, and he tipped every picture all the way going, and straightened them up on the way back! That's where I learned that if you have a problem you solve it with a sense of humour.

Chapter 12

The Moment 'Me' Returned

Edward McLaughlin

Edward McLachlin is a leading member of the Scottish Dementia Working Group, and a forthright and witty speaker at conferences. He was a painter before being diagnosed with dementia, and has kept this up but with a remarkable change of style. In this self-revelatory piece he reflects on his diagnosis and subsequent events, and their effect on his sense of playfulness.

I think humour is one of the great keys to unlocking things. In diagnosis lots of people are in a fog, a depression, a 'Why me?' syndrome. 'I've got Alzheimer's or dementia, I can't do anything, no one expects me to do anything, I'm no longer a person.'

One of the things I constantly take from this is trying to convince another person with the condition that they're still there and able to do things. It's like catching the biggest fish in the river but putting it back.

People with the best of intentions can disempower other people. What made them an individual is ripped from them. They don't realise what they're losing is their individuality.

What are we if we're not ourselves? We just become a performing puppet.

A good example is I was in a restaurant with some of the family. I was having fish and I knew that one of the family had said to the waiter, 'My father has Alzheimer's.' The waiter came up and asked, 'How's your meal? Were you happy with it?' Then he came to me and asked the same question. I answered, 'Fine.' 'Are you enjoying the fish?' I said, 'There's only one problem: it's dead.' And the idea of eating something dead on the plate swung the whole ambience of the meeting as they realised it was true of them too. It soured every meal at that table. The waiter was confused – he didn't know I was joking; it hadn't gone in the predicted direction.

Another example of black humour, and this time it was accidental. I was standing outside a house where there had been a fire, and there were police and a fire engine. The fireman came out with what was obviously a body in a body bag and carried it down to the waiting people. The woman standing next to me, a little old granny figure, asked the fireman 'Is he dead?' You'd think that with him carrying a body bag and putting it in a van to go to the mortuary the answer would be obvious. But he said, 'We're not allowed to tell you.' They locked the van door. Then she asked a policeman. He said, 'I'm sorry, madam, while there's an investigation going on we're not allowed to make any public comments.' You thought to yourself, 'Who's the person with cognition problems?'

When I got the diagnosis I didn't know what Alzheimer's was – I thought it was fatigue. I'd been too busy for years, but I wanted something from the doctor to pick me up. I said I was exhausted physically and mentally and I didn't know how to untangle myself. Eventually I ended up in hospital – I really was exhausted, I thought I'd had a heart attack.

Eventually I had these scans and the doctor said, 'You've got Alzheimer's.' They discovered I had a spastic heart, and they couldn't do anything about it. I think this is what caused the brain damage. They said, 'We want your driving licence,' and they took it and cut it up and said to the nurse, 'Send it to Cardiff.' But there was a little lightball flashing in my head because I still had my pilot's licence!

My then wife and I came home and I went back to work. My wife went back to the dementia unit where she worked. Later we sat down to discuss what was going on. I felt slightly reassured because I thought she had experience and would be coming forewarned to the situation, but I was naïve. She told me that she liked working in the area, but she couldn't live with my diagnosis. She then informed me that she'd been in a relationship for the past two years. I had been so busy earning money that I hadn't noticed.

This was the point where a dark day became pitch black. It went from confusion to hell. I was totally cut adrift. My friends took over and got me another house. I moved into a family flat and for six months I lived out of cardboard boxes that my friends had packed. Everybody in some other synopsis will go through something similar to this.

Eventually, with the help of my community psychiatric nurse, I became reconciled to the situation. It had been a painful period but I began to enjoy my new-found freedom.

Now I began to be conscious of my environment. I live in the country and I went for walks. I enjoyed the pleasure of being outside and noticing things. I walked round a corner and bumped into my old self. I'd always been an observer and I picked up where I'd left off: like a magnet I attracted things into myself.

The moment that pointed the whole thing up was when I was in the kitchen making a meal; there was a chopping board, and I was cutting up an onion. Suddenly my head was coming closer and closer to the board, and then (I couldn't stop myself) I thumped my head on it. I'd actually been walking into things for a long time without rationalising it. My depth of field had altered. It was a eureka moment. Things started to make a bizarre kind of sense. There was a tremendous relief, and humour fell back into place.

The sound of my grandchildren laughing, my friends telling me jokes – these had meant nothing to me. I couldn't react and they didn't get the expected response. Whatever the mechanism in the psyche is it didn't work: it had been stunned out of existence. For just under two years I had managed without it, and it was a sad place.

Chapter 13

Play the Game

Robin Lang

Town Break, Stirling, is a day centre celebrated for its innovative practices. Robin Lang has been a volunteer there for some years; his warmth and bonhomie are infectious, and he conveys this in his contribution.

I'm a volunteer at the Town Break, Stirling. I always used to do the door. When I open the door I always sing, usually 'You are my sunshine'. It triggers others to sing. You see them a little bit down, but when you do that the light comes on.

Now this group of men we have just now are marvellous at singing – we're a wee bit choir. In fact they've given a performance in here. Just a fortnight ago I opened the door and there they were; they immediately burst out with 'You are my sunshine' with the hands up and everything – they'd been practising in the taxi! So I just joined in with them. It's in everyone, all you have to do is give them the stimulus and they're away on their own.

And when the men are playing dominoes, and the women are playing musical bingo, often when the snatch of a tune comes up the men will sing the whole song.

You play the game with each person. Sometimes the playfulness is teasing and a wind-up. I got to know this lady and that she had been a land girl. But latterly she was from the

West End of Glasgow, and I was from the East End. Well once I'd got on her wavelength I started to send her up. I'd say, 'Oh it's Elizabeth from Kelvinside, or is it Be(tt)y from Glasgow?' (the accents I would use would suit each district). And she'd say, 'I'll sort you out!' with a clenched fist but a twinkle in her eye.

A year later, months after she'd left us, I was visiting a care home and I happened to see her: she was sitting in a chair stony-faced, the way they always are in those places. I went up to her, knelt down and caught her eye. 'Oh it's Elizabeth from Kelvinside, or is it Be(tt)y from Glasgow?' I asked. Without hesitation, 'I'll sort you out!' she said, with a twinkle in her eye, and waved her fist in the old way. Working with people with dementia is the best fun ever.

Working with them at home can be a nightmare: it's difficult to laugh when you're hurting. The carer is living with the characteristics of dementia 24/7. I don't say keeping humour in the situation is impossible but I do say it's very difficult. I reckon it would take an exceptional person to manage it in these circumstances. It is good if you can do it – there are times when if you don't laugh you would cry. I have met a few wives and husbands who were in that situation.

One thing to survive is that you must realise the person isn't necessarily doing something on purpose. Knowledge is the key to unlocking the frustration that people often feel. Even if knowledge fails there is often the option to absent yourself for a brief period.

It's quite different in the Town Break situation. Here there is no baggage – you don't share a history with the person. You are only with them for two hours at a time. Knowing a bit about the background and working life of the person is a good starting point. Then you can use it in a humorous fashion, you can play the game from the start. For example, suppose a man had worked on the platform of an engine: I would ask him 'Did you ever fry an egg on a shovel?' The answer he gave might be 'Aye, it burnt more often than not!'

I'm also a befriender, so I meet people, the same people in the group situation and on their own. I see them in the day centre and in the home. Jack is fairly crabbit (sullen) at home. The only time his wife hears him laugh is when we're playing dominoes. And when there's Joe there too and we're all competing, the opportunities for humour are even greater. Playing dominoes with me is not a silent thing. We have a pattern of play and stimulus – it's well worn. But Jack is getting less responsive, so I'll have to find a new strategy, to adapt to playfulness on a different level.

And it's only with these two that I'm like this; with others it would be different. I wouldn't try anything like that – you have to know which buttons to push.

One day Jack gets into my car and says, 'How're you feeling?' And I say, 'I'm fine.' He says, 'And how does that feel like?' He's set me up for it. It's not just what you say, it's the way that you say it, and how you look: the twinkle in the eye. And I get added humour from re-telling it to the other men, and he's there enjoying it again too.

We take groups on social outings. Imagine somebody who doesn't speak any more. A group go tenpin bowling with their family carers. To make it easier the bowl is put on a ramp and then pushed. Well this man gets a strike. He strikes a pose too, arms in the air, and shouts 'Yes!' His wife is almost in tears.

Or there's a trip on the canal. Jack has the helm, and I'm way at the back of the boat. The look on his face is amazing: he is like a wee boy in his glory. And it lasts: he has talked about it so much afterwards. Yes, it is the greatest joy seeing people have fun!

Chapter 14

Your Hat's Squint

Nicola Hodge

> *Nicola Hodge is a volunteer at Town Break, Stirling, a*
> *day centre celebrated for its innovative practices. In her*
> *remarkable piece she covers a lot of ground: caring for her*
> *father, her relationship with one attender at Town Break, a*
> *special event she organised there, and a recent visit to China.*
> *The constant thread is provided by a playful approach.*

A strange title but when you look after someone who has
dementia why be miserable? Each and every one of us is an
individual, we are all different and we enjoy fun in different
ways, so when I was asked to write about fun in dementia
I thought about the wonderful, humorous times that I have
experienced when I've been blessed to help someone with
dementia. I want to share them with you. I hope they make
you jolly.

I have a great passion for people who have dementia and
I love their stories. I was very mature and anxious when I
decided to go down the academic route, and commit myself
to study at the age of 54 – but I never looked back. Within
my sociology degree I studied dementia, not knowing that I
would eventually use that knowledge to look after my father
and help others who sadly have the most horrific illness one

can imagine – namely, to be imprisoned within your own mind.

He was a wonderful journalist, my father, and sadly he took vascular dementia. For a man of words it was difficult, but I tried to make life as interesting as possible for him. He had interviewed many important people in his life but the most memorable and exciting one was Elvis Presley. Records show that he was the only British journalist who ever interviewed and was photographed with Elvis on UK soil (*The Scotsman*, 6 June 2009). The photographs of that meeting played a very important part when reminiscing with him: the happiness and laughter we shared as he would take me back to that memorable night at Prestwick Airport when he met The King of rock 'n' roll. It was jubilant. The many care staff in his life loved to hear about that meeting and look at the photograph of the two together in famous conversation. Many times Elvis's music would be played and the staff and I would sing and dance with tears in our eyes as the laughter and fun flowed.

My father went out with joy. (Isaiah 53: 12–13)

I have been blessed in my life to be involved with a wonderful organisation called Town Break; it gives support to people and their carers in the early stages of Alzheimer's and dementia. This organisation gave me the opportunity to befriend a lady called Joy – so well named! She brought great jollity into my life. When I met Joy she had the early onset of Alzheimer's disease. She lived very independently in sheltered housing but loved company because she had travelled widely in her life and loved to share stories and pictures with anyone who wanted a blether!

I would visit her weekly for two hours in an afternoon and always looked forward to them because she was an inspirational lady who loved life and had a wonderful sense of humour, and we had fun, gaiety and laughter. Some afternoons it was feeding the ducks, visiting our favourite coffee shop or the pub and playing dominoes! However, the highlight of our meetings was always when it was a 'rainy day'. I had not known Joy very long when I discovered she loved clothes; she was a very elegant lady who had enjoyed an eclectic life. Many photographs were displayed in her home and it was when I enquired about the people and celebrations in them that Joy discovered she could take herself back and relive many of those occasions. I was also taken into a world of dressing up and glamour. Joy had a wardrobe bulging with every outfit you can imagine. Dresses, shoes, hats, gloves, jewellery and handbags that she had worn to family weddings, christenings, graduations, funerals – you name it, she had it. Such joy! When we could not go out she would dress up and she would dress me!!!! Bless, I would sit roasting when I was draped with fur, leopard skin or lace. Joy would have veils of fascinating tulle falling over her head while elegantly holding a Chanel clutch bag and endowed with pearls. She would relive her memories of the occasions, telling me every detail of who was there and what they wore, as she paraded around her sitting room dressed from head to toe in finery. We did laugh at each other. The occasion always had to finish with 'as we would have done, Nicola, no tea mugs in my day' – with an afternoon tea tray, silver teapot, fine china, linen napkins, sugar lumps and tongs. How I miss those scones!

My delightful days with Joy gave me an idea to help other people relive their dressing-up days. Town Break offers a lunch club twice a week for people to come and have fun in the cocktail bar (well, tea lounge), reminisce, have lunch, play games, sing and just be happy. I decided to relive their wedding day. I organised a wedding lunch for 30 people. It was manic! I needed a lunch menu, cake, flowers, bunting, hats, outfits, guests, music, and a bride and groom! The week before, I set the scene, and had everyone getting into the spirit of the occasion by making buttonholes, bunting and table decorations. Invitations were sent to the relatives of the clients. On the morning of the big day, the hall was transformed into a magic place of balloons, paper doilies, cake stands all standing to attention, bunting, flowers and ecstatic merriment. It had an air of festivity. The top table creaked with as many pieces of reminiscence that I could find. The local charity shops offered an array of wedding attire fit for kings and queens. If an extra hat was required, a tea cosy was at hand! I begged and borrowed food and refreshments from local shops. The volunteers all had different roles to play and we had a beautiful bride and groom dressed with Joy's approval. An added attraction was a young bride-to-be who came along for some words of wisdom from the experienced guests. The photograph albums of all the clients' weddings were on display, and the laughter of their hilarious stories lifted the roof. One client was a retired minister who spoke so eloquently it brought tears of joy. I had managed to get an archive newspaper photograph of one of the ladies' wedding day. Mary was overjoyed. We danced and sang. One lady still remembers the occasion to this day; she sang to her husband with tears of joyfulness (sadly it was to be one of her final memories of her husband).

My final story of joy in dementia is international. I talk about my love and compassion for people who have dementia but my greatest lesson came when I visited Beijing (summer 2011). I went to Beijing to teach English (proofreading a book for a Chinese gentleman) but a main reason was to see how people who had dementia were looked after in a Chinese hospital. With all the regulations connected to China it was not easy to break down barriers to allow me into a hospital, but I succeeded and was spiritually rewarded many times. I have Professor Wang of the Peking Mental Health Teaching Hospital to thank for her kindness and her wonderful team of nurses who opened their hearts to me. Oh elation when I met them all! My mandarin was sparse; I knew how to say hello and a few words of exchange and that I was from Sugelan. I soon realised that I did not need any language – I only needed to touch and smile with those wonderful people; the more I smiled, the more their smiles grew and grew wider and wider. The smiles gradually led to laughter and the joy in that hospital ward was infectious, amazing. I was shown art and embroidery all crafted with pride and dignity. They taught me how to play Chinese chequers using mandarin characters; no language was necessary – a shout when I made a correct move and a hug when I went wrong. I tried to show my British expertise with table tennis, but they had such skill, I was hopeless, but not in their eyes: the tears of joy would run down each of our faces. The day I said goodbye my question was would I ever repeat this joyousness and pleasure?

There are no barriers to hilarity – it can start with the tiniest particle within your soul and can spread into an epidemic of fun and laughter, so why should it make any difference if you have dementia? See me, not the disease. Yes I can see you, Joy – your hat's squint!

The optimist sees the rose and not its thorns; the pessimist stares at the thorns, oblivious to the rose. (Kahlil Gibran 1883–1931)

Chapter 15

Beyond Right and Wrong

Ian Cameron

Ian Cameron has over ten years' experience of the Elderflowers project, which brings episodes of hilarity to units in hospitals in Scotland, as described in Chapter 4. He shows that clowning is a special gift to people with dementia, and that providing it is a serious business.

There's really no difference from clowning in the theatre and working with people on a dementia unit. You might consider them extremes but it is to do with human communication and being playful within that.

The playfulness is what we should all be doing all the time. It is through play that we learn and make mistakes. It's an area for being able to make mistakes freely, to celebrate them and enjoy them. We don't have to be 'right'. I heard Russell Ackoff, the systems theorist, on the radio. He was talking about teaching in business and the value of mistakes. He said that if you don't make mistakes all that you learn is what you already know. School education is based on being right. If children make a mistake they are told they are wrong rather than encouraged to learn from their mistakes.

In the Elderflowers work the playful interchanges occupy a place beyond right and wrong. Yesterday there was a lady who started to say 'ukulele' and I repeated it and we began playing with the word and singing it. In a sense she gave me the word to play with. In clowning the rules might be simple; if they understand them people can join in. If the rules are difficult the game is lost. Play is not total anarchy. In the choreography of clowning you play within the rules but no two games are ever the same.

Adults can suppress their playfulness with the feeling that they must be serious. Clowns are very serious about life and always trying to do their best, but they fail and that is where the humour comes from. If a clown tries to be funny, it never works.

In the dementia units when people make a mistake and they laugh about it, you can join in their laughter: you have to be in complicity with them. We can laugh at confusion too by showing people that there's nothing wrong with it.

Music is play. At present we are trying out something called 'Musical Wash'. It's a kind of catalyst, that is light and playful in the playing. The way it works is like this: we start to play instruments outside the room, so people hear us before they see us. Then we enter the room and keep playing for about 15 minutes. There's no immediate expectation of a response. It gives time for people to see us and for us to see them, without either party doing anything specific. Then things begin to happen in their own time and playfulness begins to emerge. Yesterday there was a point where I was playing music and ladies said things to me so I mirrored them back with the harmonica. In this way I was being playful in playing the music, so the idea of playfulness was introduced before the music stopped.

People with dementia are losing the ability to control their actions: they have been put in a passive situation, and their opinions are not being asked. Working as a clown you can give them the opportunity to make judgements, the chance to regain their powers. We present simple situations like: 'We're going to a wedding. What do I need to do?' Or even more simply, going down on our knees and asking, 'What do I need to do to get up?'

I think it helps that I'm around the age of some of the younger people in the dementia units. With Elderflowers I feel I can give more than with Clown Doctors for this reason.

With every unit I go to, even if I've been there before, I feel it as a challenge. You can't expect the responses from day to day or minute to minute, you never know how people might react. It makes you open to where each person is, and that's most important. And this is in the nature of play: if you held onto set patterns it wouldn't work at all. I think there is actually a match between people with dementia and play in this – neither involves holding onto set patterns, and both rely upon responding spontaneously to what occurs.

There is a tendency for adults without the condition to seem more rule bound, and playfulness loses out. Firms send staff on courses sometimes to encourage them to re-connect with that side of themselves. Some people go a bit wild at the weekend, maybe get drunk, to counteract their weekday rule-bound lives.

Doing theatre gives me an avenue for play, and working with people with dementia gives me an extension of that: it is focusing play in different ways.

Successful engagement is to do with energy. Sometimes when you go into a room, even if you are only working with one person, you can feel the energy created spreading through the room and affecting other people. This is something staff sometimes comment on: that everyone was in a bit of a mood, and then you relaxed them.

Sometimes you come away and think: that's what it's all about. And sometimes not. But that's par for the course – it would be a miracle if our activity always worked well. Sometimes you come out of a unit and you feel you didn't quite find the right way in with someone. It is always a learning experience.

I often wonder: how long does the effect of your visit last? How long does someone remember? How is their mood changed by the visit? These are questions evaluation has to deal with but they are not easy to answer. The moment is just as important, though. And we're all like that to a certain extent. Our enjoyment is largely in the moment, doing it. The fact is we can remember it, but is that what matters most? Someone with dementia is fully engaged in the moment, which in a way is what is most significant in life. And what is most significant in art.

As an actor in a production with dialogue you learn the lines in order to forget them. People with dementia don't have to learn to forget. It is the same in physical theatre – you remember things in your body once you have learned them. Of course people with dementia sometimes remember – perhaps it is a song, but it's just like the actor who has forgotten the lines, they're still there. In the case of a song it may be the music or the words or a rhythm or all three together.

There was one woman who couldn't see very well, but she noticed colours and textures. Then she would start singing. This was always the pattern. Then one day she started telling about her past. She obviously felt safe with us. But this was after some months of visits.

You will be working with someone and you may take out an object or a postcard or sing a song and it's just right. One time around Burns Night I started reading out a poem very loud and actorly, and a lady across the room started to laugh, surfing the energy of the moment as if she'd got caught by it, and she kept on repeating the laugh – and she wasn't even the person we were working with!

Sometimes we have taken in kitchen implements and said, 'I've just bought this in a shop, and I don't know how to use it.' Some people might remember what it was used for, but others might find a new use for it or even appreciate it for itself as an object.

There was one occasion when I put fairy lights all over my head and body. They were worked with a switch. Someone suggested I was like Blackpool Tower. Then it was decided that we would have an opening of the lights. We needed someone to perform the opening ceremony. There was this lady who had been very quiet but she volunteered to do it. She made the perfect speech, I switched on the lights, and everyone clapped. I think she had been a headmistress but had never played any part in our proceedings before.

The red noses act as a sign of playfulness. There was one unit where we had told the staff what we were about in advance, gave them red noses, and they had already tried them out, so people had expectations of what we were there for when we arrived. Some staff have to be won over, some are very responsive. Some take to playfulness and others seem to see the beginning and end of sessions as the boundaries of playfulness. Some staff say, 'Your friends the Elderflowers are coming today!', put images of us up on the walls, or show them red noses in anticipation. Others say and do nothing.

To sum up, in this work you are a catalyst for releasing something – you never know what it will be, but you treasure it when it occurs. You never presume, but always keep an open mind.

References

Batson, P. (1998) 'Drama as therapy: bringing memories to life.' *Journal of Dementia Care 6*, 4, 19–21.

Bayley, J. (1998) *Iris: A Memoir*. London: Duckworth.

Benson, S. (2009) 'Ladder to the Moon: interactive theatre in care settings.' *Journal of Dementia Care 17*, 4, 20.

Breckman, R. (2000) 'Julie smiled with eyes overrunning with laughter.' *Share*, June.

Byers, A. (1995) 'Beyond marks: on working with elderly people with severe memory loss.' *Inscape 1*.

Cohen, E. (2003) *The House on Beartown Road*. New York: Random House.

Connor, J. (1997) *A Funny Thing Happened on the Way to the Nursing Home*. Ourimbah, Australia: Book Bound Publishing.

Coulman, C. (2012) 'Living life is good for us! Using laughter in care settings for older people.' *Living Life*.

Graty, C. (2008) 'Centre stage.' *Living and Dementia*, December.

Heywood, B. (1994) *Caring for Maria*. London: Element.

Killick, J. (2003) 'Funny and sad and friendly: a drama project in Scotland.' *Journal of Dementia Care 11*, 1, 24–26.

Killick, J. (2010) 'The Funshops: improvised drama and humour.' *Journal of Dementia Care 18*, 6, 14–15.

Killick, J. (2011) 'The power of laughter.' *Journal of Dementia Care 19*, 1, 13–14.

Kitwood, T. (1998) 'French connection.' *Journal of Dementia Care 6*, 4, 11.

Knocker, S. (2000) 'A meeting of worlds – play and metaphor in dementia care and dramatherapy.' Unpublished manuscript.

Knocker, S. (2010) 'The Dictator Time.' In J. Gilliard and M. Marshall (eds) *Time for Dementia*. London: Hawker Publications.

MacCaig, E. (ed.) (2005) *The Poems of Norman MacCaig*. Edinburgh: Polygon.

Nachmanovitch, S. (1990) *Free Play: Improvisation in Life and Art.* New York: Tarcher/Putnam.

Naughtin, G. and Laidler, T. (1991) *When I Grow Too Old to Dream: Coping with Alzheimer's Dissease.* North Blackburn, Australia: Collins Dove.

Perrin, T. (1997) 'The puzzling, provocative question of play.' *Journal of Dementia Care 5*, 2, 15–17.

Perrin, T. and May, H. (2000) *Wellbeing in Dementia: An Occupational Approach.* London: Churchill Livingstone.

Pulsford, D., Connor, J. and Rushforth, D. (1999) 'Does play demean people with dementia?' *Journal of Dementia Care 7*, 5, 15.

Thompson, K. (1998) 'Therapeutic clowning with people with dementia.' *Hospital Clown Newsletter 3*, 2.

Vogler, S. (2003) *Dementia: The Loss… The Love… The Laughter.* New York: 1stBooks.

West, S. (2009) Letter in *Living with Dementia*, May.

Whitehead, J. (2008) 'Laughter and Alzheimer's.' Available at www.laughteryoga.co.uk, accessed on 24 June 2012.

Wylie, K. (2001) 'Expressing her playfulness, love and laughter.' *Journal of Dementia Care 9*, 6, 22–23.

Zoutewelle-Morris, S. (2011) *Chocolate Rain: 100 Ideas for a Creative Approach to Activities in Dementia Care.* London: Hawker Publications.

Further Reading and Resources

On play

Nachmanovitch, S. (1990) *Free Play: Improvisation in Life and Art*. New York: Tarcher/Putnam.

On humour

Provine, R. (2000) *Laughter: A Scientific Investigation*. New York: Penguin Putnam.

On dementia and play

Perrin, T. and May, H. (2000) *Wellbeing in Dementia: An Occupational Approach*, Chapter 5 'The playful practitioner'. London: Churchill Livingstone.

DVDs

Red Nose Coming (film of Elderflowers). Available at www.dementiashop.co.uk/products/red-nose-coming-dvd-clowning-and-communication-care-homes, accessed on 24 June 2012.

Pop (film by Joel Meyerowitz). Available at www.pbs.org/wgbh/pages/frontline/shows/pop/etc/joel.html, accessed on 24 June 2012.

Websites

Clowning: www.heartsminds.org.uk; www.clowndoctors.com.au, accessed on 24 June 2012.

Entertainment: www.computing.dundee.ac.uk/projects/circa, accessed on 17 September 2012.

General: www.dementiapositive.co.uk, accessed on 24 June 2012.

Humour: www.deepfun.com/funflow.html, accessed on 24 June 2012.

Laughter Yoga: www.joyworks.co.uk; www.unitedmind.co.uk, accessed on 24 June 2012.

Index